BCS

Monoclonal Antibodies
and Cancer

Academic Press Rapid Manuscript Reproduction

Proceedings of the IV Armand Hammer Cancer Symposium

Monoclonal Antibodies and Cancer

Edited by

Barbara D. Boss
Rod Langman
Ian Trowbridge
Renato Dulbecco

The Salk Institute for Biological Studies
La Jolla, California

1983

ACADEMIC PRESS, INC.
(Harcourt Brace Jovanovich, Publishers)
Orlando   San Diego   San Francisco   New York   London
Toronto   Montreal   Sydney   Tokyo   São Paulo

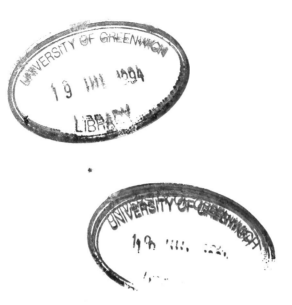

ACADEMIC PRESS, INC.
Orlando, Florida 32887

United Kingdom Edition published by
ACADEMIC PRESS, INC. (LONDON) LTD.
24/28 Oval Road, London NW1 7DX

LIBRARY OF CONGRESS CATALOG CARD NUMBER: 83-73587
ISBN 0-12-118880-9

PRINTED IN THE UNITED STATES OF AMERICA

83 84 85 86   9 8 7 6 5 4 3 2 1

Contents

Contributors   xv
Preface   xxiii

I   THERAPY

The Present

Therapeutic Trials of Monoclonal Antibody in Leukemia and Lymphoma: Biologic Considerations

Ronald Levy, Richard A. Miller, Paul T. Stratte, David G. Maloney, Michael P. Link, Timothy C. Meeker, Allan Oseroff, Kristiaan Thielemans, and Roger Warnke

   I. Introduction   5
  II. Results   7
 III. Discussion   12
      References   14
      Questions and Answers   15

Mouse Monoclonal Antibodies *in Vivo*

Hilary Koprowski

   I. Introduction   17
  II. Use of Monoclonal Antibodies in Detection of Gastrointestinal
      Cancer   18

III. Use of Monoclonal Antibodies in the Study of Human Tumor
     Heterotransplants   21
IV. Variation in the Expression of Monoclonal Antibody-Defined Antigens
     in Human Tumor Metastases   25
 V. Mouse Monoclonal Antibody Treatment of Patients with Colorectal
     Cancer   28
     Abbreviations   36
     References   36
     Questions and Answers   38

Monoclonal Antibody Therapy of Chronic Lymphocytic Leukemia and Cutaneous T-Cell Lymphoma: Preliminary Observations

Kenneth A. Foon, Robert W. Schroff, Deborah Mayer, Stephen A. Sherwin, Robert K. Oldham, Paul A. Bunn, and Su-Ming Hsu

  I. Introduction   39
 II. Materials and Methods   40
III. Results   42
IV. Discussion   49
     Abbreviations   51
     References   51

Therapeutic Potential of Monoclonal Antibodies That Block Biological Function

Ian S. Trowbridge

  I. Introduction   53
 II. Results and Discussion   54
     Abbreviations   60
     References   60
     Questions and Answers   61

Prospects for Antibody Therapy of Leukemia: Experimental Studies in Murine Leukemia

Christopher C. Badger and Irwin D. Bernstein

  I. Introduction   63
 II. Antibody Treatment of Transplanted Leukemia   64
III. Antibody Treatment of Spontaneous Leukemia   66
IV. Toxicity of Antibody Therapy   70
 V. Discussion   70
     Abbreviations   72
     References   72

Autologous Bone Marrow Transplantation for Stage IV Abdominal Non-Hodgkin's Lymphoma after *in Vitro* Purging with Anti-Y 29/55 Monoclonal Antibody and Complement

C. Baumgartner, P. Imbach, A. Luthy, R. Odavic, H. P. Wagner, G. Brun del Re, U. Bucher, H. K. Forster, A. Hirt, and A. Morell

  I. Introduction   74
 II. Materials, Methods, and Patients   74
III. Results   77
 IV. Conclusions   77
     Abbreviations   78
     References   79
     Questions and Answers   79

The Future

Magic Bullets

The Use of Immunotoxins for the Treatment of Cancer

Jonathan W. Uhr and Ellen S. Vitetta

  I. Introduction   85
 II. Results and Discussion   87
     Abbreviations   95
     References   96
     Questions and Answers   97

Immunotoxins

Hildur E. Blythman, Pierre Casellas, Olivier Gros, Franz K. Jansen, Jean-Claude Laurent, Gilbert Richer, and Hubert Vidal

  I. Introduction   99
 II. Results and Discussion   100
     Abbreviations   105
     References   105
     Questions and Answers   106

Monoclonal Antibody–Ricin Conjugates for the Treatment of Graft-versus-Host Disease: Present and Future Prospects

David M. Neville, Jr., Richard J. Youle, John H. Kersey, and Daniel A. Vallera

  I. Introduction   107
 II. Results   108

III. Discussion   110
     Abbreviations   113
     References   113
     Questions and Answers   116

Blockade of the Galactose-Binding Site of Ricin by Its Linkage to Antibody

Philip Thorpe, Alex Brown, Brian Foxwell, Christopher Myers, Walter Ross, Alan Cumber, and Tony Forrester

  I. Introduction   117
 II. Preparation of Conjugates   118
III. Fluorescence-Activated Cell Sorter Analysis of Cell Binding   119
 IV. Cytotoxicity Experiments   119
  V. Conclusion   123
     References   123
     Questions and Answers   124

Monoclonal Antibody Conjugates for Diagnostic Imaging and Therapy

Mette Strand, David A. Scheinberg, Otto A. Gansow, and A. M. Friedman

  I. Introduction   125
 II. Imaging   126
III. Therapy   127
 IV. Conclusions   130
     Abbreviations   131
     References   131
     Questions and Answers   131

Human Monoclonal Antibodies

Construction of Heteromyelomas for Human Monoclonal Antibody Production

Nelson N. H. Teng, Francisco Calvo-Riera, Kit S. Lam, and Henry S. Kaplan

  I. Introduction   135
 II. Materials and Methods   136
III. Results   138
 IV. Discussion   139
     Abbreviations   140
     References   141
     Questions and Answers   142

Human Hybridomas: Comparison of Human Cell Lines for Production of Human Hybridomas and Development of Human Hybridomas Producing Antigen-Specific IgG Using *in Vitro*-Immunized Peripheral Blood Cells as Fusing Partners

Kenneth A. Foon, Paul G. Abrams, Jeffrey L. Rossio, James A. Knost, and Robert K. Oldham

    I. Introduction   143
   II. Materials and Methods   145
 III. Results   147
 IV. Discussion   152
       Abbreviations   154
       References   154
       Questions and Answers   155

Production of Stable Human–Human Hybridomas at High Frequency

Joy G. Heitzmann and Melvin Cohn

    I. Introduction   157
   II. Results and Discussion   158
       Abbreviations   161
       References   161
       Questions and Answers   162

Human Monoclonal Antibodies to Human Cancers

Mark C. Glassy, Harold H. Handley, Ivor Royston, and D. Howard Lowe

    I. Introduction   163
   II. Materials and Methods   164
 III. Results   165
 IV. Discussion   167
       Abbreviations   170
       References   170

The Clinical Potential of Human Monoclonal Antibodies in Oncology

Karol Sikora, Thomas Alderson, and Howard Smedley

    I. Introduction   171
   II. Methods   172
 III. Results   173
 IV. Discussion   179
       Abbreviations   180
       References   180

Human–Human Hybridomas

Paul A. W. Edwards, Michael J. O'Hare, and A. Munro Neville

    I. Introduction   181
   II. Results   182
  III. Conclusions   182
       References   183

II DIAGNOSIS

Immunohistological Analysis of Human Malignancies with Monoclonal Antibodies

David Y. Mason and Kevin C. Gatter

    I. Introduction   187
   II. Materials and Methods   187
  III. Results and Discussion   188
       References   196
       Questions and Answers   197

Differential Reactivity of Monoclonal Antibodies with Human Colon Adenocarcinomas and Adenomas

Daniela Stramignoni, Robert Bowen, Jeffrey Schlom, and Barbara F. Atkinson

    I. Introduction   199
   II. Results   200
  III. Discussion   204
      Abbreviations   205
      References   205
      Questions and Answers   206

Monoclonal Antibodies Potentially Useful in Clinical Oncology

Maria Ines Colnaghi, Silvana Canevari, Gabriella Della Torre, Sylvie Mènard, Silvia Miotti, Mario Regazzoni, Elda Tagliabue, Renato Mariani-Costantini, and Franco Rilke

    I. Materials and Methods   207
   II. Results   208
     Abbreviations   213
     References   213

Clinical Significance of the Monoclonal Antibody Anti-Y 29/55, Reactive Against Human Follicular Center-Derived B Lymphocytes and Their Neoplastic Counterparts

Hansjörg K. Forster, Theo Staehelin, Jean-Paul Obrecht, and Fred G. Gudat

I. Introduction   215
II. Results   216
III. Conclusions   217
    Abbreviations   220
    References   220

The Isolation and Characterization of Monoclonal Antibodies Against Murine Alpha Fetoprotein

A. I. Goussev, A. K. Yasova, and O. M. Iezhneva

I. Introduction   223
II. Results   223
    Abbreviations   225
    References   225

Use of Antibodies to Membrane Antigens in the Study of Differentiation and Malignancy in the Human Breast

Joyce Taylor-Papadimitriou, Joy Burchell, and Sidney E. Chang

I. Introduction   227
II. Antigenic Determinants on HMFG Recognized
    by HMFG-1 and HMFG-2   228
III. Reactions with Sections of Breast Tissue and Tumors   229
IV. Reactions with Cultured Mammary Epithelial Cells   230
V. Expression of HMFG-1 Antigen and Reduced Growth
    of Normal Mammary Epithelium   232
VI. Use of HMFG Antibodies to Detect Cancer Cells *in Vivo*
    and *in Vitro*   234
VII. Comparison to Other Antibodies Recognizing Similar
    Antigenic Determinants   235
    Abbreviations   236
    References   236
    Questions and Answers   238

Differential Turnover Rate of Surface Proteins in Actively Proliferating and Differentiated C_6 Glioma Cells

Shail K. Sharma, Rakesh Kumar, and U. N. Singh

I. Introduction   239
II. C_6 Glioma Cells as a Model System in Studies on Differentiation   240
    Abbreviations   242
    References   242

HLA-DR Expression on Nonlymphoid Human Tumor Cells: Biochemical and Histochemical Studies with Monoclonal Antibodies

G. Riethmüller, J. Johnson, R. Wank, D. J. Schendel, H. Göttlinger, E. P. Rieber, and J. M. Gokel

  I. Introduction   243
 II. Monoclonal Antibody 16.23 Recognizes an Allotypic Determinant
     on the Beta Chain of HLA-DR3   244
III. *In Vivo* Expression of Ia-Like Antigens on Mammary Carcinoma Cells
     and Correlation with Infiltrating Lymphocyte Subsets   246
     Abbreviations   249
     References   249

Cancer-Associated Carbohydrate Antigens Detected by Monoclonal Antibodies

John L. Magnani and Victor Ginsburg

  I. Introduction   251
 II. A Gastrointestinal Cancer-Associated Antigen Detected by Monoclonal
     Antibody 19-9 is a Ganglioside Containing Sialylated Lacto-*N*-Fucopentaose
     II in Colorectal Carcinoma Cell Line SW 1116   251
III. Sialylated Lacto-*N*-Fucopentaose II is Present on a Mucin in Patient's
     Sera   254
 IV. Monoclonal Antibodies Directed Against the Human Le^b Blood
     Group   255
  V. Many Monoclonal Antibodies with Apparent Specificity to Human Tumors
     Are Directed Against Lacto-*N*-Fucopentaose III   255
 VI. Summary   257
     References   259
     Questions and Answers   260

Mapping of Antigenic Sites on Human Transferrin by Monoclonal Antibodies

V. Viklický, J. Bártek, H. Verlová, P. Dráber, and V. Hořejší

  I. Introduction   261
 II. Results   261
     Abbreviations   264

Application of Tumor-Localizing 791T/36 Monoclonal Antibody in Radioimmunodetection of Experimental and Human Tumors and Targeting Cytotoxic Drugs Such as Vindesine and Methotrexate

R. W. Baldwin, M. J. Embleton, and M. V. Pimm

  I. Introduction   265
 II. *In Vivo* Localization of Radioisotope-Labeled Antitumor Monoclonal
     Antibody in Human Tumor Xenografts   266

    III. Tumor Detection by External Imaging of Radionuclide-Labeled 791T/36
        Antibody   267
    IV. Drug Targeting Studies   268
    V. Conclusions   272
        Abbreviations   273
        References   273
        Questions and Answers   274

In Vitro Screening of New Monoclonal Anti-Carcinoembryonic Antigen Antibodies for Radioimaging Human Colorectal Carcinomas

Charles M. Haskell, Franz Buchegger, Magali Schreyer, Stefan Carrel, and Jean-Pierre Mach

    I. Introduction   275
    II. Materials and Methods   276
    III. Results and Discussion   276
        Abbreviations   282
        References   282
        Questions and Answers   283

Monoclonal Antibodies That Bind to Normal and Neoplastic Breast Epithelial Cells Distinguish Subsets of Normal Breast Epithelial Cells

Paul A. W. Edwards and Christopher S. Foster

    I. Introduction   285
    II. Antigenic Heterogeneity in Tumors   286
    III. Antigenic Heterogeneity in Normal Tissue   286
    IV. These Observations Can Be Generalized to Other Tissues
        and Monoclonal Antibodies   287
    V. Interpretation and Consequences   288
    VI. Conclusion   290
        References   291
        Questions and Answers   292

Index   295

Contributors

Numbers in parentheses indicate the pages on which the authors' contributions begin.

Paul G. Abrams (143), Biological Therapeutics Branch, Biological Response Modifiers Program, Division of Cancer Treatment, National Cancer Institute, Frederick Cancer Research Facility, Frederick, Maryland 21701

Thomas Alderson (171), Ludwig Institute for Cancer Research, MRC Centre, Cambridge CB2 2QH, United Kingdom

Barbara F. Atkinson (199), Department of Pathology and Laboratory Medicine, University of Pennsylvania, Philadelphia, Pennsylvania 19104

Christopher C. Badger (63), Medical Oncology and Pediatric Oncology Programs, Fred Hutchinson Cancer Research Center, and Departments of Medicine and Pediatrics, University of Washington, Seattle, Washington 98104

R. W. Baldwin (265), Cancer Research Campaign Laboratories, University of Nottingham, Nottingham NG7 2RD, United Kingdom

J. Bártek (261), Czechoslovak Academy of Sciences, Institute of Molecular Genetics, Prague, Czechoslovakia

C. Baumgartner (73), Department of Pediatrics, University Hospitals, Inselspital, 3010 Bern, Switzerland

Irwin D. Bernstein (63), Medical Oncology and Pediatric Oncology Programs, Fred Hutchinson Cancer Research Center, and Departments of Medicine and Pediatrics, University of Washington, Seattle, Washington 98104

Hildur E. Blythman (99), Centre de Recherches Clin-Midy, 34082 Montpellier, France

Robert Bowen (199), Laboratory of Tumor Immunology and Biology, National Cancer Institute, National Institutes of Health, Bethesda, Maryland 20205

Alex Brown (117), Imperial Cancer Research Fund, London WC2A 3PX, United Kingdom

G. Brun del Re (73), Central Hematology Laboratory, University Hospitals, Inselspital, 3010 Bern, Switzerland

Franz Buchegger (275), Department of Biochemistry, University of Lausanne, Lausanne, Switzerland

U. Bucher (73), Central Hematology Laboratory, University Hospitals, Inselspital, 3010 Bern, Switzerland

Paul A. Bunn (39), Clinical Oncology Program, Division of Cancer Treatment, National Cancer Institute, Frederick Cancer Research Facility, Frederick, Maryland 21701

Joy Burchell (227), Imperial Cancer Research Fund, London WC2A 3PX, United Kingdom

Francisco Calvo-Riera (135), Cancer Biology Research Laboratory, Department of Radiology, Stanford University School of Medicine, Stanford, California 94305

Silvana Canevari (207), Division of Experimental Oncology A, Istituto Nazionale Tumori, Milano, Italy

Stefan Carrel (275), Ludwig Institute for Cancer Research, Epalinges Sur/Lausanne, Switzerland

Pierre Casellas (99), Centre de Recherches Clin-Midy, 34082 Montpellier, France

Sidney E. Chang (227), Imperial Cancer Research Fund, London WC2A 3PX, United Kingdom

Melvin Cohn (157), Developmental Biology Laboratory, The Salk Institute for Biological Studies, La Jolla, California 92037

Maria Ines Colnaghi (207), Division of Experimental Oncology A, Istituto Nazionale Tumori, Milano, Italy

Alan Cumber (117), Chester Beatty Research Institute, London, United Kingdom

P. Dráber (261), Czechoslovak Academy of Sciences, Institute of Molecular Genetics, Prague, Czechoslovakia

Paul A. W. Edwards (181, 285), Ludwig Institute for Cancer Research (London Branch), Royal Marsden Hospital, Sutton, Surrey SM2 5PX, United Kingdom

M. J. Embleton (265), Cancer Research Campaign Laboratories, University of Nottingham, Nottingham NG7 2RD, United Kingdom

Kenneth A. Foon (39, 143), Biological Therapeutics Branch, Biological Response Modifiers Program, Division of Cancer Treatment, National Cancer Institute, Frederick Cancer Research Facility, Frederick, Maryland 21701

Tony Forrester (117), Chester Beatty Research Institute, London, United Kingdom

Hansjörg K. Forster (73, 215), Central Research Units, F. Hoffmann-La Roche and Co. Ltd., CH-4002 Basel, Switzerland

Christopher S. Foster (285), Ludwig Institute for Cancer Research (London Branch), Royal Marsden Hospital, Sutton, Surrey SM2 5PX, United Kingdom

Brian Foxwell (117), Imperial Cancer Research Fund, London WC2A 3PX, United Kingdom

A. M. Friedman (125), Chemistry Division, Argonne National Laboratory, Argonne, Illinois 60439

Otto A. Gansow (125), Department of Chemistry, Michigan State University, East Lansing, Michigan 48824

Kevin C. Gatter (187), Nuffield Department of Pathology, University of Oxford, United Kingdom

Victor Ginsburg (251), National Institute of Arthritis, Diabetes, and Digestive and Kidney Diseases, National Institutes of Health, Bethesda, Maryland 20205

Mark C. Glassy (163), Cancer Center, Department of Medicine, University of California, San Diego, La Jolla, California 92093

J. M. Gokel (243), Pathology Institute, University of Munich, Munich, Federal Republic of Germany

H. Göttlinger (243), Institute for Immunology, University of Munich, Munich, Federal Republic of Germany

A. I. Goussev (223), Laboratory of Tumor Immunochemistry and Immunodiagnosis, Cancer Research Centre, Moscow, USSR

Olivier Gros (99), Centre de Recherches Clin-Midy, 34082 Montpellier, France

Fred G. Gudat (215), Institute of Pathology, University of Basel, CH-4002 Basel, Switzerland

Harold H. Handley (163), Cancer Center, Department of Medicine, University of California, San Diego, La Jolla, California 92093

Charles M. Haskell (275), Cancer Center, Medical Research Services, VA West Los Angeles, and Department of Medicine, School of Medicine, University of California, Los Angeles, Los Angeles, California 90073

Joy G. Heitzmann (157), Developmental Biology Laboratory, The Salk Institute for Biological Studies, La Jolla, California 92037

A. Hirt (73), Institute for Clinical and Experimental Cancer Research, Tiefenauspital, 3004 Bern, Switzerland

V. Hořejší, (261), Czechoslovak Academy of Sciences, Institute of Molecular Genetics, Prague, Czechoslovakia

Su-Ming Hsu (39), Laboratory of Pathology, Division of Cancer Biology and Diagnosis, National Cancer Institute, National Institutes of Health, Bethesda, Maryland 20205

O. M. Iezhneva (223), Laboratory of Tumor Immunochemistry and Immunodiagnosis, Cancer Research Centre, Moscow, USSR

P. Imbach (73), Department of Pediatrics, University Hospitals, Inselspital, 3010 Bern, Switzerland

Franz K. Jansen (99), Centre de Recherches Clin-Midy, 34082 Montpellier, France

J. Johnson (243), Institute for Immunology, University of Munich, Munich, Federal Republic of Germany

Henry S. Kaplan (135), Cancer Biology Research Laboratory, Department of Radiology, Stanford University School of Medicine, Stanford, California 94305

John H. Kersey (107), Department of Therapeutic Radiology and Laboratory of Medicine/Pathology, University of Minnesota, Minneapolis, Minnesota 55455

James A. Knost (143), Biological Therapeutics Branch, Biological Response Modifiers Program, Division of Cancer Treatment, National Cancer Institute, Frederick Cancer Research Facility, Frederick, Maryland 21701

Hilary Koprowski (17), The Wistar Institute, Philadelphia, Pennsylvania 19104

Rakesh Kumar (239), Department of Biochemistry, All India Institute of Medical Sciences, New Delhi-110029, India

Kit S. Lam (135), Cancer Biology Research Laboratory, Department of Radiology, Stanford University School of Medicine, Stanford, California 94305

Jean-Claude Laurent (99), Centre de Recherches Clin-Midy, 34082 Montpellier, France

Ronald Levy (5), Department of Medicine, Stanford University, Stanford, California 94305

Michael P. Link (5), Department of Medicine, Stanford University, Stanford, California 94305

D. Howard Lowe (163), Department of Surgery, University of California, San Diego, La Jolla, California 92093

A. Luthy (73), Department of Pediatrics, University Hospitals, Inselspital, 3010 Bern, Switzerland

Jean-Pierre Mach (275), Ludwig Institute for Cancer Research, Epalinges Sur/Lausanne, Switzerland

John L. Magnani (251), National Institute of Arthritis, Diabetes, and Digestive and Kidney Diseases, National Institutes of Health, Bethesda, Maryland 20205

David G. Maloney (5), Department of Medicine, Stanford University, Stanford, California 94305

Renato Mariani-Costantini (207), Division of Anatomical Pathology and Cytology, Istituto Nazionale Tumori, Milano, Italy

David Y. Mason (187), Nuffield Department of Pathology, University of Oxford, United Kingdom

Deborah Mayer (39), Biological Response Modifiers Program, Division of Cancer Treatment, National Cancer Institute, Frederick Cancer Research Facility, Frederick, Maryland 21701

Timothy C. Meeker (5), Department of Medicine, Stanford University, Stanford, California 94305

Sylvie Mènard (207), Division of Experimental Oncology A, Istituto Nazionale Tumori, Milano, Italy

Richard A. Miller (5), Department of Medicine, Stanford University, Stanford, California 94305

Silvia Miotti (207), Division of Experimental Oncology A, Istituto Nazionale Tumori, Milano, Italy

A. Morell (73), Institute for Clinical and Experimental Cancer Research, Tiefenauspital, 3004 Bern, Switzerland

Christopher Myers (117), Imperial Cancer Research Fund, London WC2A 3PX, United Kingdom

A. Munro Neville (181), Ludwig Institute for Cancer Research (London Branch), Royal Marsden Hospital, Sutton, Surrey SM2 5PX, United Kingdom

David M. Neville, Jr. (107), Section on Biophysical Chemistry, Laboratory of Neurochemistry, National Institute of Mental Health, National Institutes of Health, Bethesda, Maryland 20205

Jean-Paul Obrecht (215), Department of Internal Medicine, University Clinics, Kantonal Hospital, CH-4002 Basel, Switzerland

R. Odavic (73), Department of Pediatrics, University Hospitals, Inselspital, 3010 Bern, Switzerland

Michael J. O'Hare (181), Ludwig Institute for Cancer Research (London Branch), Royal Marsden Hospital, Sutton, Surrey SM2 5PX, United Kingdom

Robert K. Oldham (39, 143), Biological Therapeutics Branch, Biological Response Modifiers Program, Division of Cancer Treatment, National Cancer Institute, Frederick Cancer Research Facility, Frederick, Maryland 21701

Allan Oseroff (5), Department of Medicine, Stanford University, Stanford, California 94305

M. V. Pimm (265), Cancer Research Campaign Laboratories, University of Nottingham, Nottingham NG7 2RD, United Kingdom

Mario Regazzoni (207), Division of Experimental Oncology A, Istituto Nazionale Tumori, Milano, Italy

Gilbert Richer (99), Centre de Recherches Clin-Midy, 34082 Montpellier, France

E. P. Rieber (243), Institute for Immunology, University of Munich, Munich, Federal Republic of Germany

G. Riethmüller (243), Institute for Immunology, University of Munich, Munich, Federal Republic of Germany

Franco Rilke (207), Division of Anatomical Pathology and Cytology, Istituto Nazionale Tumori, Milano, Italy

Walter Ross (117), Chester Beatty Research Institute, London, United Kingdom

Jeffrey L. Rossio (143), Biological Therapeutics Branch, Biological Response Modifiers Program, Division of Cancer Treatment, National Cancer Institute, Frederick Cancer Research Facility, Frederick, Maryland 21701

Ivor Royston (163), Cancer Center, Department of Medicine, University of California, San Diego, La Jolla, California 92093

David A. Scheinberg (125), Department of Pharmacology and Experimental Therapeutics, The Johns Hopkins University School of Medicine, Baltimore, Maryland 21205

D. J. Schendel (243), Institute for Immunology, University of Munich, Munich, Federal Republic of Germany

Jeffrey Schlom (199), Laboratory of Tumor Immunology and Biology, National Cancer Institute, National Institutes of Health, Bethesda, Maryland 20205

Magali Schreyer (275), Ludwig Institute for Cancer Research, Epalinges Sur/Lausanne, Switzerland

Robert W. Schroff (39), Biological Response Modifiers Program, Division of Cancer Treatment, National Cancer Institute, Frederick Cancer Research Facility, Frederick, Maryland 21701

Shail K. Sharma (239), Department of Biochemistry, All India Institute of Medical Sciences, New Delhi-110029, India

Stephen A. Sherwin (39), Biological Response Modifiers Program, Division of Cancer Treatment, National Cancer Institute, Frederick Cancer Research Facility, Frederick, Maryland 21701

Karol Sikora (171), Ludwig Institute for Cancer Research, MRC Centre, Cambridge CB2 2QH, United Kingdom

U. N. Singh (239), Molecular Biology Unit, Tata Institute of Fundamental Research, Bombay-400005, India

Howard Smedley (171), Ludwig Institute for Cancer Research, MRC Centre, Cambridge CB2 2QH, United Kingdom

Theo Staehelin (215), Central Research Units, F. Hoffmann-La Roche and Co. Ltd., Ch-4002 Basel, Switzerland

Daniela Stramignoni (199), Laboratory of Tumor Immunology and Biology, National Cancer Institute, National Institutes of Health, Bethesda, Maryland 20205

Mette Strand (125), Department of Pharmacology and Experimental Therapeutics, The Johns Hopkins University School of Medicine, Baltimore, Maryland 21205

Paul T. Stratte (5), Department of Medicine, Stanford University, Stanford, California 94305

Elda Tagliabue (207), Division of Experimental Oncology A, Istituto Nazionale Tumori, Milano, Italy

Joyce Taylor-Papadimitriou (227), Imperial Cancer Research Fund, London WC2A 3PX, United Kingdom

Nelson N. H. Teng (135), Cancer Biology Research Laboratory, Department of Radiology, Stanford University School of Medicine, Stanford, California 94305

Kristiaan Thielemans (5), Department of Medicine, Stanford University, Stanford, California 94305

Philip Thorpe (117), Imperial Cancer Research Fund, London WC2A 3PX, United Kingdom

Gabriella Della Torre (207), Division of Experimental Oncology A, Istituto Nazionale Tumori, Milano, Italy

Ian S. Trowbridge (53), Cancer Biology Laboratory, The Salk Institute for Biological Studies, La Jolla, California 92037

Jonathan W. Uhr (85), Department of Microbiology, University of Texas Health Science Center, Dallas, Texas 75235

Daniel A. Vallera (107), Department of Therapeutic Radiology and Laboratory of Medicine/Pathology, University of Minnesota, Minneapolis, Minnesota 55455

H. Verlová (261), Czechoslovak Academy of Sciences, Institute of Molecular Genetics, Prague, Czechoslovakia

Hubert Vidal (99), Centre de Recherches Clin-Midy, 34082 Montpellier, France

V. Viklický (261), Czechoslovak Academy of Sciences, Institute of Molecular Genetics, Prague, Czechoslovakia

Ellen S. Vitetta (85), Department of Microbiology, University of Texas Health Science Center, Dallas, Texas 75235

H. P. Wagner (73), Department of Pediatrics, University Hospitals, Inselspital, 3010 Bern, Switzerland

R. Wank (243), Institute for Immunology, University of Munich, Munich, Federal Republic of Germany

Roger Warnke (5), Department of Medicine, Stanford University, Stanford, California 94305

A. K. Yasova (223), Laboratory of Tumor Immunochemistry and Immunodiagnosis, Cancer Research Centre, Moscow, USSR

Richard J. Youle (107), Section on Biophysical Chemistry, Laboratory of Neurochemistry, National Institute of Mental Health, National Institutes of Health, Bethesda, Maryland 20205

Preface

For several years, annual symposia sponsored by Dr. Armand Hammer have been held at the Salk Institute to bring together leading investigators in basic and clinical cancer research to discuss new advances in this field. A major goal of these symposia has been to catalyze the development of practical applications in cancer from basic research in cell biology and immunology. Since the hybridoma technique was first described by Köhler and Milstein in 1975, monoclonal antibodies have opened up a wealth of new possibilities in the treatment and diagnosis of cancer. For this reason, and because of the extraordinarily rapid progress made in this area in the last few years, monoclonal antibodies in cancer was chosen for the topic of the fourth Armand Hammer Symposium.

This volume, based on the proceedings of the 1983 symposium, was produced in order that a critical and comprehensive review of the uses of monoclonal antibodies in cancer be available to a wider audience. The topics discussed range from the present status of clinical trials of monoclonal antibodies in the treatment of leukemia and solid tumors and the use of monoclonal antibodies in the diagnosis and detection of tumors, to the development of human monoclonal antibodies, as well as new approaches to monoclonal antibody therapy including experimental studies with cytotoxic antibody–toxin conjugates or "magic bullets." This volume will be of interest to the clinician or basic investigator wishing to know about the latest developments in monoclonal antibody research in relationship to cancer. It will also be valuable to experts in the field as it contains a wealth of previously unpublished data.

The topics covered in this book have been organized into two sections dealing with therapeutic and diagnostic applications of monoclonal antibodies in cancer. The order of contributions to these sections has been arranged so that those describing applications of monoclonal antibodies that have already progressed to clinical trials appear first, followed by articles dealing with studies that form the basis for new ways to exploit monoclonal antibodies in cancer in the future.

We hope that this book will not only provide the reader with a current account of the rapidly developing field of monoclonal antibodies in cancer, but also transmit the excitement and optimism of investigators in the field generated by the present use of monoclonal antibodies in diagnosis and treatment of cancer and sustained by even greater prospects for the future.

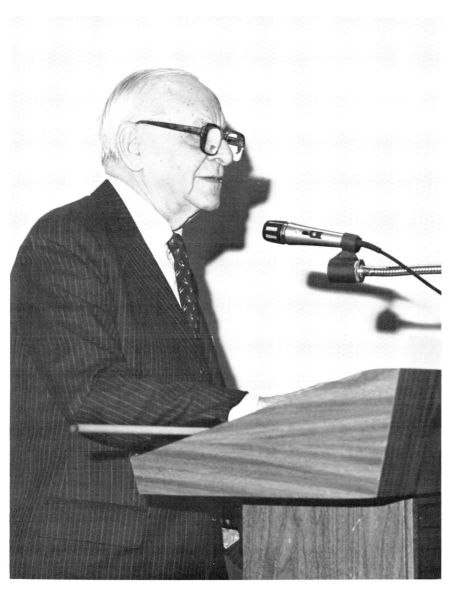

Dr. Armand Hammer, President of The Armand Hammer Foundation, at the opening of the IV Armand Hammer Cancer Symposium on January 12, 1983.

THERAPY   I

The Present

THERAPEUTIC TRIALS OF MONOCLONAL ANTIBODY IN LEUKEMIA AND LYMPHOMA: BIOLOGIC CONSIDERATIONS[1]

Ronald Levy, Richard A. Miller, Paul T. Stratte,
David G. Maloney, Michael P. Link,
Timothy C. Meeker, Allan Oseroff,
Kristiaan Thielemans and Roger Warnke

Department of Medicine
Stanford University
Stanford, California

I. INTRODUCTION

At this second annual conference on monoclonal antibodies and cancer it is important to compare and update our clinical and experimental results, analyze our successes and perceived problems and chart a course for future work. In this presentation, we will restrict our attention to a consideration of mouse monoclonal antibodies administered directly to patients with malignancy. Other contributors will deal with the subjects of human monoclonal antibodies, drug-toxin conjugates and treatment of bone marrow with antibodies in vitro for the purpose of autologous transplantation.

The majority of the clinical trials with monoclonal antibodies to date have been done in patients with leukemia and lymphoma. We will rely primarily on examples from our own trials and amplify on these when appropriate using results of other groups. In all cases, the patients in these initial studies had exhausted conventional therapies. In Table 1 are listed what we consider to be some of the facts that have

[1]This work was supported by grants CA 21223, CA 05838 and CA 33399 from the National Institute of Health and grant IM 114 from the American Cancer Society.

emerged so far from the clinical studies with monoclonal antibodies. To begin with, mouse monoclonal antibodies can be
administered safely in man by the intravenous route in doses
as high as 800mg. Toxicity has been limited to fever, chills,
anaphalactoid reactions and dyspnea. All of these side
effects can be avoided by slow infusion rates and by premedi-
cation with antipyretics and antihistamines. Other routes of
administration, antibody formulations and schedules must still
be examined. Nevertheless, the lack of serious toxicity will
give considerable license to future studies which will employ
monoclonal antibodies in clinical settings of lower tumor
burdens (which may prove more responsive to biological therapies).

TABLE 1.   Facts about Monoclonal Antibodies as Cancer
            Therapeutic Agents

---

1. Mouse antibody can be administered safely in man.
    a. Doses: Up to 800mg.
    b. Routes: I.V., slowly infused. Others?

2. Antitumor effects can be observed.
    a. Usually of short duration.
    b. Limited to leukemia and lymphoma?

3. Mouse monoclonal antibodies are immunogenic in man.
    a. Anti-idiotype is part of the response.
    b. Implication : or human antibodies?

4. Monoclonal antibodies can induce antigenic modulation.
        Possible solutions:
            Schedule of antibody administration.
            Monovalent antibody.
            Nonmodulating antigens.

5. Monoclonal antibodies do not kill cells directly.
        What are the relative roles of:
            Complement?
            Antibody-dependent cell-mediated cytotoxicity?
            Reticuloendothelial system?

TABLE 2. **Anti-Leu-1** Monoclonal Antibody: Mycosis
Fungoides/Cutaneous T Cell Lymphoma

Pt	Total Dose (mg)	Number of Treatments	Treatment Duration (Days)	Toxicity	Anti-Mouse	Measurable Tumor Response
RC	2	2	2	Fever Chills	No	N.E.
L	164	17	75	None	No	P.R.
CI	102	9	31	Cutaneous Pain and Edema	Yes	P.R.
G	761	14	57	None	Yes	P.R.
DH	151	16	66	None	Yes	P.R.
MG	106	13	35	Respiratory Distress	No	M.R.
FC	13	4	13	N.E.	N.E.	N.E.
AIK	378	6	17	Myalgias Fever Urticaria	Yes	N.R.
GG	54	8	27	Fever Urticaria	No	M.R.

N.E. = Not Evaluable, P.R. = Partial Remission, M.R. =
Minimal Response, N.R. = No Response, Pt = Patient

with toxicity such as allergy or immune complex disease, even
though the administration of mouse Ig was continued. However,
when it occurred, the anti-mouse antibody blocked the therapeutic effect of the mouse monoclonal. An example of this is
shown in Figure 2, where the elimination of circulating Sezary
cells by mouse monoclonal antibody was progressively reduced
by the appearance of anti-mouse antibody. We have dissected
this immune response and found that it is directed primarily
against the constant region determinants of the mouse Ig mole-

II. RESULTS

Antitumor effects have been documented in man.
ranged from transient reductions in circulating leu!
to sustained and clinically significant regressions
tumor masses. Tables 2 and 3 summarize our result
groups of patients: those with cutaneous T cell lyr
those with acute lymphocytic leukemia of T cell type
former group, a single monoclonal antibody, anti-Le
used (1). In the latter group, two other antibodi
investigated in addition to anti-Leu-1. None of tl
bodies in either of these two studies were absolutel
for the tumor cells since they also react with normal
ocytes. That antitumor effects can be achieved usi
bodies which are not tumor specific was predicted
experiments of Bernstein and his collaborators (2).
other hand, the most impressive clinical result was
using an antibody with a high degree of tumor specifi
anti-idiotype antibody directed against the surface
B cell lymphoma (Figure 1) (3). This patient achieve
plete clinical remission which has lasted for over a
a half without any other therapy. This was despite t
that he had progressive lymphoma unresponsive to conv
chemotherapy prior to treatment with the monoclonal a1
A discussion of the mechanism of the antitumor effe
below.

Mouse monoclonal antibodies are immunogenic in ma
our initial studies we administered aggregate-free, ul
trifuged globulin preparations in the hope that they
induce immunoglobulin tolerance (4). However, we hav
cluded that the failure of some patients to respond t
mouse Ig is due to a general immunoincompetence second
their underlying disease or to prior therapies. Ma
patients, as well as normal subhuman primates, produc
anti-mouse Ig antibody response. We have not been abl
prevent this response by deaggregating the globulin o
administering cyclophosphamide along with the antibo
Interestingly, we found that when an unreactive mouse
myeloma protein was infused into a chimpanzee, no imm
response occurred. However, when the same chimp was s1
quently challenged with the T cell reactive anti-Leu-1
body, an anti-mouse response was produced, albeit a blu
one (5). In patients the immune response was not assoc:

TABLE 3. Monoclonal Antibody Trials: T Cell Acute Lymphocytic Leukemia

Pt	Antibody	Total Dose (mg)	Number of Treatments	Treatment Duration (Days)	Toxicity	Anti-Mouse	Transient Reduction of Circulating Cells	Sustained Tumor Response
TW	17F12	129	34	19	Sporadic Coagulation Defect	None	Yes	No
SB	17F12 12E7	20 10	3	6	None	N.D.	Yes	No
JW	4H9 17F12 12E7	25 25 50	4	4	None	N.D.	No	No
JSa	17F12 4H9 12E7	50 40 50	4 3 4	11	None	N.D.	N.A.	No
SN	4H9	20	1	1	None	None	No	No
JSp	17F12 12E7 4H9	325 475 100	11 13 2	42	Fever Chills	Yes	Yes	Yes

N.D. = Not Done, N.A. = Not Applicable, Pt = Patient.

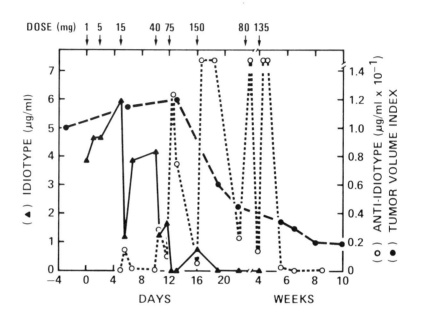

FIGURE 1.   In Vivo Effects of Anti-Idiotype.   Levels of
serum idiotype (triangles) and anti-idiotype (open circles)
are indicated over the course of therapy.   The tumor response
to anti-idiotype therapy is represented by the plot of tumor
volume index (solid circles).   Reproduced with permission.

cule.   However, a small, but significant, fraction of the
antibodies produced are directed against the combining site,
or idiotype, of the monoclonal.   These anti-idiotype antibodies completely block the interaction between the monoclonal
antibody and its antigen in vitro.   When human monoclonal
antibodies become available for clinical trials, it will be
important to determine if they too will evoke an anti-
idiotypic immune response.
      Monoclonal antibodies induce antigenic modulation which
can be an important mechanism of tumor escape in vivo (6).
This was first shown by Ritz and colleagues with the anti-
CALLA antibody (7).   Subsequently, we have observed antigenic
modulation to a variable degree in all the patients we have
treated with the anti-Leu-1 monoclonal antibody.   It is

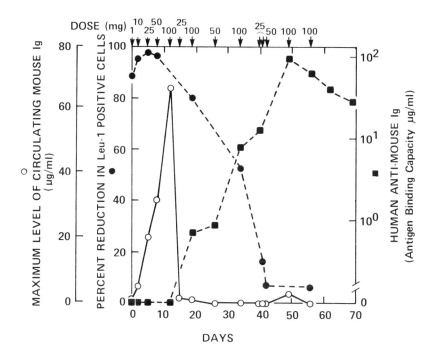

FIGURE 2. Anti-Mouse Antibody Response by a Patient Treated with Anti-Leu-1. Doses of antibody and schedule of administration are shown at the top. Reduction in circulating lymphoma cells at the end of each dose (solid circles). Level of mouse antibody achieved in the serum at the end of each dose (open circles). Anti-mouse antibody (solid squares).

somewhat surprising that monoclonal antibodies can induce antigenic modulation, especially of an antigen like Leu-1, which has only one antigenic site per molecule. In this case, extensive cross-linking and lattice formation on the cell surface is difficult to imagine. Several approaches have been suggested to deal with this problem in therapy, including scheduling antibody administration in such a way as to allow for reappearance of the target on the cell (8), constructing monovalent antibodies (9) and choosing nonmodulating antigens.

Finally, one must come to a consideration of the mechanism responsible for antitumor effects of monoclonal antibodies in vivo. From numerous experimental systems it can be concluded that serum complement plays, if anything, only a minor role in this process (2, 10-13). Instead, a number of cellular effector systems have been implicated (9-11). Our clinical results indicate that the antibody-coated cells in vivo are ultimately the limiting factors in the antitumor effect. In those patients who have not made anti-mouse antibody, tumor cells eventually escape destruction due to an exhaustion of the effector cell system. This is true despite continued administration of the monoclonal antibody and adequate coating of the antigen-positive tumor cells in vivo (8). However, when we analyzed the case of the B cell lymphoma patient who responded so dramatically to treatment with an anti-idiotype antibody, we found an extensive infiltrate of reactive T cells and macrophages in and around the tumor cells in the regressing lymph nodes. It may be that, in addition to being so specific for the tumor (14), anti-idiotype antibodies are a special case in which host control of normal B cell proliferation can be evoked for the B cell tumor. In the future, therefore, we will need to search for antibodies for other types of tumors which not only bind with a degree of specificity but are able to affect cell proliferation either through direct effects on the tumor cells or through a recruitment of normal regulatory controls.

III. DISCUSSION

We are left with a number of important questions to answer before we can decide about the ultimate role of monoclonal antibodies in the therapy of human malignancy. Some of these questions are listed in Table 4. As regards the issue of antibody specificity, it seems that for therapy, as opposed to diagnosis, absolute tumor specificity may not be required. The key question is how to improve the potency of antibodies in eliminating tumor cells. If a cellular effector system is involved, can it be enhanced? If not, can it be by-passed by making the antibodies intrinsically toxic to cells by coupling drugs or toxins to them? Most intriguing seems to be the postulate that antigenic targets may exist which are involved in the regulation of cell growth and that antibodies against

such targets may prove more efficacious. Next to these questions, the issues of immunogenicity, antibody class and tissue
penetration are secondary and certainly answerable in the
foreseeable future.

TABLE 4. Questions About Monoclonal Antibodies as Cancer
          Therapeutic Agents

---

1. Can absolute tumor specificity be achieved?
      Is it necessary?

2. Can the potency of antibodies be improved?
   a. Combining with toxic substances.
   b. Enhancement of in vivo systems for elimination of
      antibody-coated cells.
   c. Antigen targets involved in regulation of cell growth.

3. Can the immune response against antibodies be avoided?
   a. Human antibodies.
   b. Specific tolerance.
   c. Reduction of immunogenicity.

4. Is antibody class important?

5. Can antibodies penetrate tissues?
   a. Intravascular versus extravascular tumor.
   b. Poorly perfused tumors.
   c. Sanctuary sites.

Although there are clearly some promising results, it is
also clear that we are at a very early stage in the process of
exploration of a new therapeutic modality. The hope is that
we can find a role for monoclonal antibodies in the therapy of
human malignant disease. If we do, it will be because we
consider the biology of these diseases, the host-tumor interaction and the proper use of the therapies that are currently
available.

REFERENCES

1. Engleman, E.G., Warnke, R., Fox, R.I., Dilley, J.,
    Benike, C.J., and Levy, R. Proc. Natl. Acad. Sci. 78,
    1791 (1981).
2. Bernstein, I.D., Tam, M.R., and Nowinski, R.C. Science
    207, 68 (1980).
3. Miller, R.A., Maloney, D.G., Warnke, R., and Levy, R.
    New Eng. J. Med. 306, 517 (1982).
4. Dresser, D. and Gowland, G. Nature 203, 733 (1964).
5. Stratte, P.T., Miller, R.A., Amyx, H.L., Asher, D.M. and
    Levy, R. J. Biol. Resp. Mod. 1, 137 (1982).
6. Boyse, E.A., Stockert, E. and Old, L.J. Proc. Natl.
    Acad. Sci. 58, 954 (1967).
7. Ritz, J., Pesando, J.M., Sallan, S.E., Clavell, L.A.,
    Notis-McConarty, J., Rosenthal, P., and Schlossman, S.F.
    Blood 58, 141 (1981).
8. Miller, R.A. and Levy, R. Lancet, August 1, 226 (1981).
9. Glennie, M.J. and Stevenson, G.T. Nature 295, 712
    (1982).
10. Kirch, M.E. and Hammerling, U. J. Immunol. 127, 805
    (1981).
11. Herlyn, D.M., Steplewski, Z., Herlyn, M.F., and
    Koprowski, H. Cancer Res. 40, 717 (1980).
12. Shin, H.S., Hayden, M., Langley, S., Kaliss, N., and
    Smith, M.R. J. Immunol. 114, 1255 (1975).
13. Lanier, L.L., Babcock, G.F., Raybourne, R.B.,
    Arnold, L.W., Warner, N.L. and Haughton, G. J. Immunol.
    125, 1255 (1980).
14. Stevenson, G.T., Elliot, E.V., and Stevenson, F.K. Fed.
    Proc. 36, 228 (1977).

QUESTIONS AND ANSWERS

RITZ: Regarding the experiment in which a monoclonal anti-
Leu-1 was injected into a monkey and resulted in an immune
response against the murine immunoglobulin, have you found
similar results with antibodies reactive with monkey cells
other than T cells?

LEVY: We have not done any experiments yet which would answer
this question.

MELCHERS: What effect did the anti-T cell monoclonal have on
the general immune system?

LEVY: At first, we suspected there might be an immunosuppression because we did not see an immune response. Later we
found that there was an immune response to the mouse antibody
and the monoclonal antibody was not very potent.   However,
when we start using immunotoxins this question of immunosuppression may be much more critical.

MACH: Have you ever radiolabeled the monoclonal antibody that
you inject into the patient to determine the percentage of
injected antibody localized in the tumor?

LEVY: We have not done this type of study.   However, I understand the general experience is that most intact antibody ends
up in the reticuloendothelial system and immunoglobulin fragments localize better.   I might add that we ultracentrifuge
the antibody to remove aggregates and improve localization but
this does not completely solve the problem.

FOON: Have you been able to detect the injected anti-Leu-1
bound to cells associated with skin lesions in cutaneous
T cell lymphoma patients?

LEVY: We tried hard to do the localization on biopsies taken
at the end of infusion using peroxidase-labeled antibody.   It
was difficult to be convinced that any anti-Leu-1 was present.
We tend to believe that there has been some modulation in
antigen expression, indicating that the antibody reached its
target, but the argument is indirect.   In other words, adding
more anti-Leu-1 to the biopsy did not result in significant
binding.

CHEN: I wonder if you could elaborate further on the possible
regulatory effect of the anti-idiotype in the context of idio-

typic networks where the host may have established a new
steady-state suppression of the tumor.

LEVY: We spent quite some time trying to assess whether the
idiotype or anti-idiotype should be used. There was no clear
concensus, so we took the more classical approach and used the
anti-idiotype.

UHR: Have you considered the possibility that an immune response to the mouse Ig bound to the tumor cells has tipped the
balance in favor of the host? You have emphasized that the
host serum antibody response to mouse Ig can block the therapeutic effect of the mouse monoclonals. However, in the
patient with the prolonged remission, perhaps a T cell
response to the foreign antigen, mouse Ig, was effective in
killing tumor cells and thus allowing other host responses
(e.g., anti-tumor Ig idiotype) to hold the tumor cells in
check.

LEVY: It is conceivable, but this patient made no humoral
response against the mouse protein and we have not measured
any cellular activities.

LENNOX: In your systems, do univalent fragments of monoclonal
antibodies give antigenic modulation?

LEVY: There is some confusion. For example, it has been
reported in the mouse thymus-leukemia system that univalent
fragments do work, although we have always found bivalency to
be essential for modulation.

RIETHMULLER: With regard to the reaction mechanism of anti-
idiotype therapy, does the patient mount a delayed-type hyper-
sensitivity response to mouse F(ab)-idiotype or to his own
Ig-idiotype by skin test?

LEVY: No.

KAR: Can you elaborate on your method of tolerization to
mouse Ig?

LEVY: We infuse 1 to 5mg of ultracentrifuged monoclonal antibody of the same class.

MOUSE MONOCLONAL ANTIBODIES IN VIVO[1]

Hilary Koprowski

The Wistar Institute
36th and Spruce Streets
Philadelphia, Pennsylvania

I. INTRODUCTION

This paper describes data obtained firsthand in our laboratory from in vivo studies with the antitumor monoclonal
antibodies listed in Table 1. Essentially, all of these
monoclonal antibodies bind to cells of gastrointestinal tract
cancer (GIC) (1). One monoclonal antibody 16-B-13, also binds
to cells of adenocarcinoma of lung and breast, but not to
other tumors and/or normal cells (2). Two monoclonal antibodies, 19-9 and 52a, are of IgG1 isotype (3), and the three
others are IgG2a (4). The determinant recognized by the 19-9
and 52a monoclonal antibodies is the sialylic acid terminal of
a glycolipid, the sialyl-lacto-N-pentaosyl II-ganglioside (5).
The protein antigen that reacts with the 17-1A monoclonal
antibody has not been identified. The C_420-32 monoclonal
antibody immunoprecipitates antigenic structures of GIC of
M_r 180K [carcinoembryonic antigen (CEA)], 160K, 50K (normal
colon mucosa antigen) and 40K (6). Finally, 16-B-13 recognizes a protein antigen of M_r 37K extracted from the three
species of tumors listed.

---

[1]This work was supported in part by grants CA-10815, CA-21124,
CA-25874 and RR-05540 from the National Institutes of Health.

TABLE 1. Mouse Monoclonal Antibodies Used in This Study

Mice Immunized With	Code	Isotype	Specificity	Antigen
	19-9; 52a	IgG1	GIC	Sialyl-lacto-N-fucopentaosyl II-ganglioside
CRC	17-1A	IgG2a	GIC	Protein ?
	$C_4$20-32	IgG2a	GIC	180K, 160K, 50K, 40K*
Lung Adeno-carcinoma	16-B-13	IgG2a	GIC Lung Ca Breast Ca	37K

CRC = Colorectal Cancer; GIC = Gastrointestinal Cancer; Ca = Cancer.
*180K etc. refers to protein of M_r 180,000 etc.

II. USE OF MONOCLONAL ANTIBODIES IN DETECTION OF GASTRO-INTESTINAL CANCER

The ganglioside that contains the carbohydrate sialyl-lacto-N-fucopentaose II (see Table 1) is found in extracts of either primary or metastatic tumors of colon, pancreas and stomach and also in meconium, but not in extracts of normal tissue (5). This gastrointestinal cancer antigen (GICA) can easily be located in gastrointestinal cancer cells by mono-clonal antibody 19-9 in the immunoperoxidase staining reaction (Figure 1) (7). This method enables the in situ detection of GICA expression by cells of organs, which could not be obtained in quantitative assays such as radioimmuno-assay (RIA) or enzyme-linked immunosorbent assay (ELISA). Using this technique, it has been possible to detect

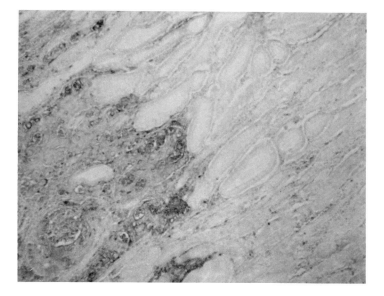

FIGURE 1. A section of gastric mucosa reacted with 19-9 antibody in a biotin-avidin immunoperoxidase procedure shows normal gastric epithelium (the pale, clear cells on the right) and dark brown stained tumor cells on the left. This gastric carcinoma is arising in and invading the normal mucosa (240x magnification).

GICA on a single layer of cells of columnar epithelium of secretory ducts such as pancreatic, hepatic, and others (Figure 2) (7).

As GICA is secreted by tumor cells, the binding of monoclonal antibodies to GICA can be used to detect this antigen in the blood of patients with gastrointestinal cancer. Using two types of assays (8), the antigen was detected in the serum of about 70-80% of patients with cancer of the pancreas and 50% of patients with either stomach or colon cancer. Whereas the GICA carbohydrate on tumor cells is linked to a ganglioside, in the serum of patients it is linked to a mucin (9). Since the mucin contains other carbohydrate chains in addition to sialyl-lacto-N-fucopentaose II, monoclonal antibodies directed against other carbohydrate determinants may enhance considerably the detection of tumor-associated antigen in the sera of cancer patients (9).

GICA is a sialylated Lewis A (Le[a]) antigen, the sialic acid being linked with the terminal sugar sequence by a still

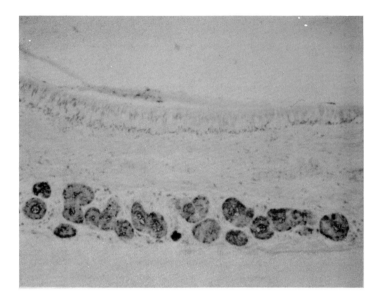

FIGURE 2. A section of bronchus of normal lung shows a dark brown reactivity of the 19-9 antibody in the immuno-peroxidase procedure with the secretory bronchial glands (across the bottom of the field), but no reactivity with the bronchial lining epithelial cells (the row of cells across the top of the field) (120x magnification).

unidentified sialyl transferase (10). The carbohydrate struc-ture of GICA is:

$$\text{NeuNAc}\alpha2\text{--}\rangle3\text{Gal}\beta1\text{--}\rangle3\text{GlcNAc}\beta1\text{--}\rangle3\text{Gal}\beta1\text{--}\rangle4\text{Glc}\beta1$$
$$4$$
$$\uparrow$$
$$\alpha1$$
$$\text{Fuc}$$

and the carbohydrate structure of Lewis A antigen is:

$$Gal\beta1--\rangle3GlcNAc\beta1--\rangle3Gal\beta1--\rangle4Glc\beta1$$
$$4$$
$$\uparrow$$
$$\alpha1$$
$$Fuc$$

The relationship between Lewis phenotype and expression of GICA is of interest. The fucosyltransferases, which are specified by the Le gene, catalyze the synthesis of sugar sequences of the Le^a antigen (see above) and of the Lewis B (Le^b) antigen, the carbohydrate structure of which is:

$$Gal\beta1--\rangle3GlcNAc\beta1--\rangle3Gal\beta1--\rangle4Glc\beta1$$
$$2 \qquad\qquad 4$$
$$\uparrow \qquad\qquad \uparrow$$
$$\alpha1 \qquad\quad \alpha1$$
$$Fuc \qquad\quad Fuc$$

In the case of the Le^b antigen, two fucosyltransferases are active. One places fucose in the 1–2 position at the terminal galactose, and the other places fucose in the 1–4 position at the 3 glucose. The first enzyme is involved in the synthesis of Le^b antigen, but not Le^a, whereas the second enzyme is required for the synthesis of both Le^a and Le^b antigens.

As shown in Table 2, there is a complete correlation between Le^{a+} subjects as determined by the presence of Le^a antigen in saliva and of GICA in saliva. On the other hand, a fraction of Le^{b+} individuals excrete GICA in saliva, probably because of competition between the sialyl transferase (which places neuraminic acid at the terminal galactose) and the fucosyltransferase (which in the Le^b phenotype places the fucose at the same position).

III. USE OF MONOCLONAL ANTIBODIES IN THE STUDY OF HUMAN TUMOR HETEROTRANSPLANTS

Human tumor cells maintained in culture will form solid tumors when implanted in nude mice (11). It is also possible to maintain progressive growth of human tumor heterotransplants in thymectomized, lethally irradiated mice reconstituted by bone marrow transplantation (12).

TABLE 2. Correlation Between Lewis Phenotype and Secretion of 19-9 GICA in Saliva

Lewis Phenotype	Normal Subjects		Cancer Patients					
			Colon Ca 19-9		Pancreas Ca 19-9		Total	
	+	−	+	−	+	−	+	−
Le^{a+b-}	6*	0	6**	0	1**	0	7	0
Le^{a-b+}	0	14*	5**	15*	0	7**	5	22
Le^{a-b-}	0	5*	0	7*	0	3*	0	11

GICA = Gastrointestinal cancer antigen; Ca = cancer.
  * = 19-9 antigen not detected in serum
 ** = 19-9 antigen present in serum

A. Imaging

Monoclonal antibodies against tumor-associated antigen(s) can be labeled with either ^{131}I or ^{125}I and used to localize human tumor heterotransplants in immunosuppressed mice. Figure 3 shows a gamma scintigraph of an immunosuppressed mouse bearing 7- to 8-day-old human GIC heterotransplants in the left flank and injected with 60-100μCi (4.6-18μg) of ^{131}I-labeled F(ab')$_2$ fragments of anti-GIC monoclonal antibody 17-1A (see Table 1). A positive tumor image can be observed in the mouse injected with the specific antibody. In comparison, mice injected with a monoclonal antibody specific for a different type of tumor will not image the GIC, and human tumors other than GIC are not imaged if an anti-GIC monoclonal antibody is used (results not shown) (13). The F(ab')$_2$ fragments of monoclonal antibody were found to show greater selectivity and specificity for human tumor heterografts in mice than intact antibody. An explanation for this might be that intact monoclonal antibodies bind Fc receptor-bearing cells in addition to tumor cells. Another factor that may contribute is that the F(ab')$_2$ fragments are cleared from blood at a significantly faster rate than intact IgG (13).

Mice bearing tumor xenografts received comparatively large doses of radiolabeled monoclonal antibody; nevertheless, administration of 200-500μg of F(ab')$_2$ fragments containing

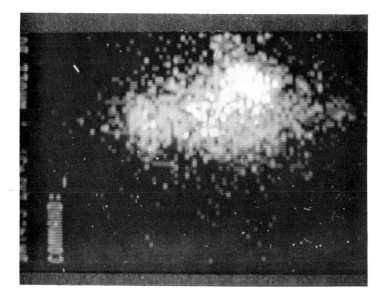

FIGURE 3. Gamma scintigraphy in tumor-bearing mouse injected three days before with 60–100µCi (4.6–18µg) of ^{131}I-labeled 17-1A F(ab')$_2$. The mouse, which was implanted with colorectal cancer in the left flank, was imaged with a parallel-hole collimator. Tumor weight was determined to be 110mg after imaging.

1–2mCi resulted in good localization of metastases of GIC in human subjects (14). In other studies, Chatal et al. (15) were able to detect 81% of GIC sites using intact monoclonal antibody and often without recourse to the background subtraction method. Moldofsky et al. (16) also studied six patients with metastasis of colon cancer who received F(ab')$_2$ fragments of monoclonal antibody 17-1A labeled with ^{131}I. In all of these patients, tumor sites became visible up to 72 hours after injection of monoclonal antibody; and, at least in one case, the liver metastasis was only 2cm in diameter. Again, tumor sites were visible without background subtraction.

B. Tumoricidal Effects

Human tumors implanted in immunosuppressed mice can be destroyed by treatment with monoclonal antibody. However, of the twenty-nine monoclonal antibodies assayed for tumoricidal properties, only seven displayed this activity. All seven were of the IgG2a isotype (Table 3). None of the monoclonal antibodies of other isotype classes showed tumoricidal effects (11).

TABLE 3. IgG2a Monoclonal Antibodies Display a Tumoricidal Effect on Xenografts of Human Tumors in Immunosuppressed Mice

| Isotype of MAb | Ratio of Monoclonal Antibodies Destroying Human Tumors | | |
	CRC	Melanoma	Lung Carcinoma
IgM	0/3	0/1	
IgA	0/1		
IgG3		0/2	
IgG2b		0/2	
IgG1	0/5	0/8	
IgG2a	4/4	2/2	1/1

CRC = Colorectal carcinoma
MAb = Monoclonal antibody

It was shown that the destruction of the tumor was not mediated by complement (11), and it has become quite obvious that monoclonal antibody mediates the tumoricidal effect by interaction with effector cells. Since the tumoricidal effect of monoclonal antibody was inhibited after injecting tumor-bearing mice with silica, the effector cell that exhibits a

tumor-suppressive effect in the presence of monoclonal antibody was identified as the macrophage (11). The monoclonal
antibody-macrophage interaction is mediated by interaction
with Fc receptors, as F(ab')$_2$ fragments of a tumoricidal monoclonal antibody are inactive. The tumoricidal effect is
highly specific as tumors are only destroyed by monoclonal
antibodies that bind specifically (Table 4). For example,
16-B-13 monoclonal antibody binds to lung, colon and breast
adenocarcinoma and mediates destruction of xenografts of these
tumors in mice, but not of melanomas which do not bind this
monoclonal antibody. The two anti-melanoma monoclonal
antibodies both show anti-human DR specificity and destroy
melanomas expressing DR antigen. On the other hand, one of
these monoclonal antibodies has no effect on Hep 2 xenografts
even though this epidermoid carcinoma also expresses DR
specificity.

The tumoricidal effect in immunosuppressed mice can be
easily reproduced in vitro by interaction of mouse peritoneal
macrophages with the respective monoclonal antibodies. Tumor
cells exposed to this mixture of monoclonal antibodies are
destroyed in tissue culture (11), as evidenced by complete
inhibition of colony formation in agar.

Mouse IgG2a monoclonal antibody also interacts with human
monocytes/macrophages after they are maintained for several
days in tissue culture (Table 5). What is interesting is the
selective development of an Fc receptor only for mouse IgG2a
by human macrophages. Human macrophages obtained from human
tumors, unlike freshly separated cells from buffy coat, also
show the presence of Fc receptors for mouse IgG2a monoclonal
antibody. This interaction permits specific destruction of
human tumors in tissue culture (Table 5) (17).

IV. VARIATION IN THE EXPRESSION OF MONOCLONAL ANTIBODY-DEFINED ANTIGENS IN HUMAN TUMOR METASTASES

In the future, when immunotherapy of tumors with monoclonal antibodies may become an established procedure, it will
be necessary to investigate antigenic variations of tumor
metastases in relation to their time and site of appearance.
A panel of monoclonal antibodies reactive with tumor cells can
be used to study this problem. Results of preliminary studies
with two tumors, gastric cancer and melanoma, are shown in
Tables 6 and 7. The binding patterns of four monoclonal
antibodies [three of which are directed against glycolipid
antigens (GICA, Le^b and Le^x) and one against the protein

TABLE 4. Inhibition of Human Tumor Xenografts in Mice by IgG2a Monoclonal Antibodies

Mice Immunized With:	Binding Specificity of MAb	MAb	Human Tumors Implanted Into Nude Mice	Ratio of Mice With Suppressed Tumor Growth
CRC	GIC	17-1A	CRC-1	54/54
			CRC-2	4/4
			MEL-1	0/5
			LC	0/8
			BC	0/5
			PC	0/5
		C414-72	CRC-1	12/12
			MEL-1	0/5
			PC	0/5
		C420-32	CRC-1	11/11
			MEL-1	0/4
			PC	0/5
		CEA*	CRC-2	7/7
LC	LC,CRC,BC	16-B-13	LC-1	5/5
			LC-2	5/5
			CRC	4/4
			BC	5/5
			MEL-1	0/5
			MEL-3	0/5
MEL	MEL (DR-antigen)	37-7	MEL-1	6/6
			MEL-2	4/4
			MEL-3 (DR-)	0/5
			EC	0/5
			CRC	0/5
		B228-8	MEL-1	5/5

CRC = Colorectal carcinoma   BC = Breast carcinoma
GIC = Gastrointestinal   EC = Hep 2 epidermoid carcinoma
         carcinoma   LC = Lung carcinoma
MEL = Melanoma   PC = Pancreas carcinoma
MAb = Monoclonal antibody
*Carcinoembryonic antigen MAb from Dr. Schlom.

TABLE 5. Interaction Between Mouse IgG2a Monoclonal Antibody and Human Monocytes/Macrophages (M/M)

Source of M/M Cells	Days in Culture	Percentage M/M Cells Expressing Fc Receptor for IgG2a MAb	Percentage Tumor Cells Releasing [^{3}H]Thymidine After Interaction With M/M and Mouse IgG2a
Blood*	29	90	87
	34	90	86
Tumor	1	50	15
	3	70	18

*From normal donors
MAb = monoclonal antibody

antigen 17–1A] to gastric cancer metastases, to liver, and to bone were determined (7). As shown in Table 6, metastases to liver shared the same binding pattern with monoclonal antibodies as the primary stomach cancer. However, cells of the bone metastases failed to bind the monoclonal antibody which defines the GICA glycolipid. Thus, in this case, there is a distinct possibility that antigenic variation occurred in the bone metastasis. This did not occur with metastases of melanoma during an 18–month observation period of another patient. As shown in Table 7, cells of melanoma metastasizing to the skin of the patient showed, in general, similar binding patterns in RIA of four monoclonal antibodies representing four different specificities. It is thus possible that metastases to the same site as the primary tumor retain antigenic characteristics of the primary tumor, whereas those metastasizing to more remote sites such as bone, undergo antigenic variation. However, it is difficult to draw any firm conclusion from a comparison of two entirely different tumors in this very preliminary study.

TABLE 6.   Variation   in   the   Expression   of   Monoclonal
           Antibody-Defined   Antigens   by   Metastases   of
           Gastric Carcinoma

TUMOR		Binding* of MAbs to Tissue Specimens:			
Site	Time Since Primary Lesion (Months)	17-1A	GICA	Le^b	Le^x
Stomach (Primary)		$\pm$	++	++	++
Liver	0	$\pm$	++	++	++
Bone	2	$\pm$	-	++	++

*In immunoperoxidase assay
MAbs = monoclonal antibodies

V. MOUSE MONOCLONAL ANTIBODY TREATMENT OF PATIENTS WITH COLORECTAL CANCER

To date, twenty patients with advanced carcinoma of the gastrointestinal tract have received one dose of mouse mono-clonal antibody along with or without buffy coat leukocytes (18,19). Extensive evaluation of the laboratory data obtained in the course of this study has been possible in thirteen patients.

A. Persistence of Mouse IgG in Serum of Patients Treated With Mouse Monoclonal Antibody

Circulating mouse IgG can be detected within a half hour after its administration to the patient and its highest levels are observed between 1-24 hours later. From then on the level of mouse IgG in those patients who received less than 133mg of monoclonal antibody (Figure 4a) decreases sharply, reaching a

TABLE 7. Variation in the Expression of Monoclonal Antibody-Defined Antigens by Metastases of Melanoma

TUMOR		Binding* to Tissue Specimens of MAb of Anti-Melanoma Group			
Site	Time Since Primary Lesion (Months)	I	II	III	VII(DR)
	Primary	2040	2350	5890	5980
	9	2720	2020	6300	4310
Skin	16	1120	2000	5660	2540
	18	1570	2330	2220	2830

*In radioimmunoassay expressed as cpm
MAb = monoclonal antibody

plateau at 8-9 days. Small amounts of mouse IgG are sometimes detected as late as 13-28 days after its administration. All patients in this group developed an anti-mouse antibody response.

In contrast, as shown in Figure 4b, the level of mouse IgG in sera of three patients who received more than 400mg of monoclonal antibody was considerably higher than that shown in Figure 4a. In the patients who received 400 and 444mg of monoclonal antibody, respectively, the circulating mouse IgG could still be detected 50-60 days later. Neither of these two patients developed an anti-mouse antibody response. Following administration of 675mg, the initial level of circulating IgG was high but it then dropped more rapidly than in the two patients mentioned above. This patient developed an anti-mouse antibody response.

Persistence of mouse IgG in patient serum did not always relate to the dose of monoclonal antibody administered, as shown by the examples illustrated in Figure 4c. Circulating mouse IgG was detected in two patients receiving either 15mg

or 366mg of monoclonal antibody for almost the same brief
period, even though the initial levels of mouse IgG were higher in the serum of the patient who received the larger dose.
In marked contrast, mouse IgG in patients who received 433mg
of monoclonal antibody circulated in the blood for longer than
fifty days at levels much higher than in the two other cases.
Neither of the two patients who received the larger doses of
monoclonal antibody developed anti-mouse antibodies, thus
ruling out the possibility that marked differences in the
levels and persistence of mouse IgG in their blood can be
attributed only to an immune response to the mouse protein.

Actual concentrations of mouse IgG in blood 24 hours after
administration of monoclonal antibody are shown in Table 8.
These values were calculated through the comparison of concentrations of mouse IgG in a patient's serum dilution to a standard dilution curve of known mouse IgG concentration in a
monoclonal antibody. The concentrations of mouse IgG observed
within 24 hours after monoclonal antibody administration, when
they are highest (Figure 4a and 4b), vary from 1.00–2.50µg/ml
of blood and do not seem to be directly related to the amount
of monoclonal antibody given. The sample, however, is so
small that it is difficult to draw definite conclusions as to
the absolute values of mouse IgG concentrations in the
patient's blood.

FIGURE 4. Panels a–c: Rabbit anti-mouse IgG antibody was
exposed to patient's serum (diluted 1:10 in buffer) and the
binding was detected by ^{125}I-labeled rabbit anti-mouse F(ab')$_2$
immunoglobulin. Panel d: Anti-colon carcinoma activity of
mouse immunoglobulin in patient's serum. Colon carcinoma
cells were incubated with patient's serum (undiluted) and
binding was determined by ^{125}I-labeled rabbit anti-mouse
F(ab')$_2$ immunoglobulin. Panel e: Presence of human antibodies against mouse immunoglobulin in patient's serum. Mouse
monoclonal anti-colon carcinoma antibody was exposed to
patient's serum (diluted 1:10 in buffer) and binding was
detected by ^{125}I-labeled goat antibodies against human F(ab')$_2$
fragments.

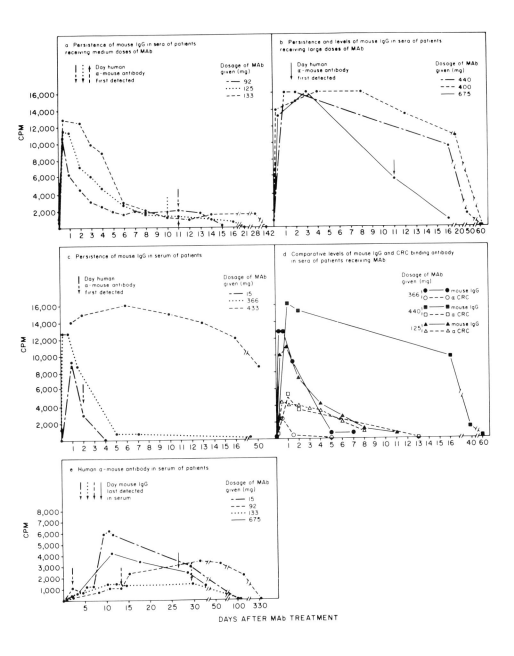

TABLE 8. The Amount of Mouse IgG Found in Serum of
          Patients

Amount of MAb Administered (mg)	MAb Concentration (µg/ml) in Blood
92	1.24
125	2.50
133	1.00
366	2.50

*Within 24 hours after administration of MAb
MAb = monoclonal antibody

B. Comparative Levels of Mouse IgG and GIC Binding
    Antibody in Sera of Patients

As shown in Figure 4d, those fractions of monoclonal antibody that bind specifically to colorectal cancer (CRC) cells
circulate in blood of patients at much lower concentrations
and for much shorter times than the mouse IgG. There is little, if any, correlation between the levels and time of persistence of mouse IgG versus its CRC binding fraction. For
instance, the anti-CRC fractions of mouse IgG present in sera
of two patients who received 125 and 440mg of monoclonal antibody, respectively, showed similar patterns of persistence,
yet there were marked differences in the levels and duration
of mouse IgG circulation in blood of the same two cases.

C. Dosage of Mouse Monoclonal Antibody and Human Anti-
    Mouse Antibody Response

As shown in Table 9, all seven patients who received less
than 137mg of mouse monoclonal antibody developed an anti-
mouse antibody response. In contrast, when the dosage of
monoclonal antibody per patient exceeded 366mg, only one of

six patients developed this response. This patient received the highest amount of mouse monoclonal antibody (675mg). Thus, the 'tolerizing dose' of mouse monoclonal antibody, if tolerance is the phenomenon involved, may lie somewhere between 350–500mg of monoclonal antibody per adult individual.

TABLE 9. Correlation Between Dosage of Monoclonal Antibody and Human Anti–Mouse Antibody Response

Amount of Mouse MAb Given (mg) In Single Injection	Ratio of Patients Developing Human Anti–Mouse Ab
15–137	7/7
366–675	1*/6

*Patient who received 675mg
MAb = monoclonal antibody

As shown in Figure 4e, the anti–mouse antibody is first detected in human serum within 2–6 days after administration of monoclonal antibody and the peak response is observed between the 8th–14th day after monoclonal antibody treatment. Human anti–mouse antibodies are detected in sera of patients for a rather long time period, usually exceeding 100 days after monoclonal antibody administration. Anti–mouse antibodies in patients who received 92mg of monoclonal antibody (Figure 4e) persisted at the same level for a period of 330 days. The earliest antibody response was observed in two patients: one who received the smallest dose of antibody (15mg) and the other who received the largest dose (675mg). In general, however, the pattern of antibody response was similar in all patients who developed such a response.

D. Response of Patients With Advanced Colorectal Cancer to Immunotherapy With Monoclonal Antibody

The data presented in Table 10 (19) refer to six patients who were treated with mouse monoclonal antibody 17–1A (see Table 1) more than five months ago and who suffered colorectal cancer metastases. Administration of even large single doses

TABLE 10. Response of Six Patients With Advanced Colorectal Cancer to Immunotherapy With Monoclonal Antibody (MAb)

MAb (mg)	Site of Metastasis	Pre-Antibody Treatment	Operation	Post-Antibody Treatment	Current Status	Observation Time (Months)	CEA ng/ml
15	Pelvic	None	Colostomy*	None	Alive with lung metastasis (18 months)	24+	1.7 Pre NC Post MAb
92	Liver	Chemo. Radiation	Liver* Resection	None	Alive with liver metastasis (8 months)	12+	17.3 Pre 1.6 30d 2.6 60d 2.9 90d 7.7 180d
125	Lung Local	Chemo.	Thoracotomy	None	A&W NED	12+	5 Pre >2.5 Since
133	Local Retroper.	None	Colostomy*	Radiation	A&W NED	9+	25 Pre >2.5 Since
366	Peritoneal	Chemo.	Laparatomy	None	A&W NED	6+	4.5 Pre >2.5 Since
400	Lung Liver	None	Biopsy Only	Chemo.	A&W**	5+	144.8 Pre 30.8 60d 12.5 90d

A&W = Alive and Well
NED = No evidence of disease
NC = No change

*Within 24 hours after administration of MAb.
**Liver and lung metastasis decreased on chest X-ray and CAT scan.

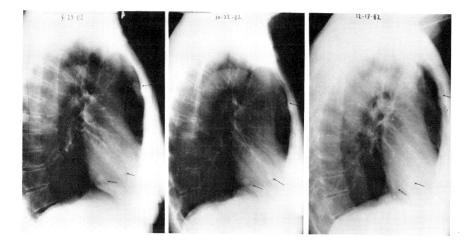

FIGURE 5. Three lateral roentgenograms demonstrating
multiple pulmonary metastases (arrows). The left frame was
obtained before the patient received monoclonal antibody. The
middle frame is two months after treatment with monoclonal
antibody and the right frame is four months after treatment.
Direct measurements demonstrate continuous (greater than 50%)
reduction in tumor size.

of mouse monoclonal antibody caused no immediate or delayed
ill effects. Surgical interventions were performed in four
patients within 24 hours after administration of monoclonal
antibody. Four of the six patients are alive and well 5–12
months after receiving immunotherapy and show either no
evidence of disease or, as in the patient who received 400mg
of monoclonal antibody, a marked decrease in the liver and
lung metastases on X-ray and computerized axial tomography
scan (Figure 5). In addition, the levels of CEA in those four
patients have consistently decreased after immunotherapy. One
of the four patients received radiation therapy and another
received drugs after treatment with monoclonal antibody. Two
patients, however, had no other treatment after immunotherapy.
Two of the patients who received smaller doses of monoclonal
antibody (15 and 92mg) had no reactivation of disease for 18
and 8 months after immunotherapy without any other treatment.
They subsequently underwent either operative resection or
radiation therapy and are alive at 12 and 24 months,
respectively, after initiation of immunotherapy.

ACKNOWLEDGMENTS

A major cooperative effort is presented in this study. Drs. Zenon Steplewski and Meenhard Herlyn produced the hybridomas and Dr. Alonzo Ross characterized the antigen defined by monoclonal antibody. Dr. Dorothee Herlyn studied imaging in mice, immunological aspects of tumoricidal effects of monoclonal antibodies in mice and levels of mouse IgG and antimouse antibodies in humans. Dr. Steplewski investigated the interaction of human macrophages with monoclonal antibodies. Dr. Barbara Atkinson of the University of Pennsylvania is in charge of immunohistological studies. Drs. John Magnani and Victor Ginsburg of NIH determined the structure of GICA and its relationship to Lewis antigen(s). Dr. Henry Sears of the Institute of Cancer Research in Philadelphia is in charge of the clinical investigations. The author thanks them for their gracious cooperation.

ABBREVIATIONS

GlC, gastrointestinal cancer; CEA, carcinoembryonic antigen; GICA, gastrointestinal cancer antigen; RIA, radioimmunoassay; ELISA, enzyme-linked immunosorbent assay; Le[a], Lewis A; Le[b], Lewis B; CRC, colorectal cancer.

REFERENCES

1. Herlyn, M., Steplewski, Z., Herlyn, D. and Koprowski, H. Proc. Natl. Acad. Sci. USA 76, 1438 (1979).
2. Mazauric, T., Mitchell, K.F., Letchworth, G.J. III, Koprowski, H. and Steplewski, Z. Cancer Res. 42, 150 (1982).
3. Koprowski, H., Steplewski, Z., Mitchell, K., Herlyn, M., Herlyn, D. and Fuhrer, P. Somat. Cell Genet. 5, 957 (1979).
4. Herlyn, D. and Koprowski, H. Proc. Natl. Acad. Sci. USA 79, 4761 (1982).
5. Magnani, J.L., Brockhaus, M., Smith, D.F., Ginsburg, V., Blaszczyk, M., Mitchell, K.F., Steplewski, Z. and Koprowski, H. Science 212, 55 (1981).
6. Blaszczyk, M., Pak, K., Lindgren, J., Pessano, S., Herlyn, M., Steplewski, Z. and Koprowski, H. Cancer Res. (submitted for publication).

7. Atkinson, B.F., Ernst, C.S., Herlyn, M.., Steplewski, Z.,
    Sears, H.F. and Koprowski, H.   Cancer Res. 42, 4820
    (1982).

8. Herlyn, M., Sears, H.F., Steplewski, Z. and Koprowski, H.
    J. Clin. Immun. 2, 135 (1982).

9. Magnani, J., Steplewski, Z., Koprowski, H. and
    Ginsburg, V. (Abstract) Fed. Proc. 42, #7, 2096 (1983).

10. Magnani, J., Nilsson, B., Brockhaus, M., Zopf, D.,
    Steplewski, Z., Koprowski, H. and Ginsburg, V. J. Biol.
    Chem. 257, 14365 (1983).

11. Herlyn, D., Steplewski, Z., Herlyn, M. and Koprowski, H.
    Cancer Res. 40, 717 (1980).

12. Herlyn, D., Atkinson, B. and Koprowski, H. J. Immunol.
    Methods 57, 155 (1983).

13. Herlyn, D., Powe, J., Alavi, A., Mattis, J., Herlyn, M.,
    Ernst, C., Vaum, R. and Koprowski, H. Cancer Res. 43,
    2731 (1983).

14. Mach, J.P., Chatal, J-F., Lumbroso, J.D., Buchegger, F.,
    Forni, M., Ritschard, J., Berche, C., Douillard, J-Y.,
    Carrel, S., Herlyn, M., Steplewski, Z. and Koprowski, H.
    Cancer Res., in press (1983).

15. Chatal, J.F., Saccavini, J.C., Fumoleau, P., Bardy, A.,
    Douillard, J., Aubry, J. and Le Mevel, B. J. Nucl. Med.
    23, 8 (1982).

16. Moldofsky, P.J. Radiology J., in press (1983).

17. Steplewski, Z., Herlyn, D., Maul, G. and Koprowski, H.
    Hybridoma 2, 1 (1983).

18. Sears, H., Atkinson, B., Mattis, J., Ernst, C.,
    Herlyn, D., Steplewski, Z., Hayry, P. and Koprowski, H.
    Lancet, April 3, 762 (1982).

19. Sears, H., Herlyn, D., Steplewski, Z. and Koprowski, H.
    JAMA (submitted for publication).

QUESTIONS AND ANSWERS

OLDHAM: What was the immunoreactivity of injected antibody in the human studies (i.e., the proportion of specific antibody to total protein)?

KOPROWSKI: Higher than in serum, but I don't know the exact figures offhand.

GUPTA: Besides macrophages, does complement play any role in antibody-dependent cytotoxic effects?

KOPROWSKI: There is no complement involvement.

OLDHAM: Have you done biopsies of responding tumors to look for antibody and/or macrophages in tumors of man and/or mouse?

KOPROWSKI: That would be a superb direct test. We are trying to work this out.

MACH: In the tumor protection experiment in nude mice, how many days after tumor challenge do you inject the monoclonal antibody? In other words, can you destroy an already growing tumor by the injection of monoclonal antibody?

KOPROWSKI: Antibody is given when there is a palpable tumor.

MONOCLONAL ANTIBODY THERAPY OF CHRONIC
LYMPHOCYTIC LEUKEMIA AND CUTANEOUS T-CELL
LYMPHOMA: PRELIMINARY OBSERVATIONS[1]

Kenneth A. Foon, Robert W. Schroff, Deborah Mayer,
Stephen A. Sherwin, and Robert K. Oldham

Biological Response Modifiers Program
Division of Cancer Treatment
National Cancer Institute
Frederick Cancer Research Facility
Frederick, Maryland

Paul A. Bunn

Clinical Oncology Program
Division of Cancer Treatment
National Cancer Institute
Frederick Cancer Research Facility
Frederick, Maryland

Su-Ming Hsu

Laboratory of Pathology
Division of Cancer Biology and Diagnosis
National Cancer Institute
Bethesda, Maryland

I. INTRODUCTION

Numerous investigators have studied the antitumor effects
of passive administration of heteroantisera (1,2). In some

---

[1]Supported in part by a DHHS Grant under contract number NO1-
CO-23910 with Program Resources, Inc.

animal studies, antiserum treatment has clearly led to inhibition of tumor growth in vivo (1). In man, similar antitumor effects of heterologous antisera have been reported, although the effects have been short-lived (1-3). More recently, monoclonal antibodies have been used in animal model systems and for treatment of human solid tumors, leukemias, and lymphomas (4-13). In general, these studies have demonstrated that monoclonal antibodies can be administered safely and evidence for an antitumor effect can be demonstrated (14,15). However, to date, most of these studies have consisted of only 2-4 patients, and a careful phase I trial has not been reported. At the National Cancer Institute, we initiated a phase I monoclonal antibody therapy trial for patients with chronic lymphocytic leukemia (CLL) and cutaneous T-cell lymphoma (CTCL). We have chosen to study the murine-derived (IgG_{2a}) T101 monoclonal antibody (16) that identifies a 65,000 molecular weight antigen (T65) found on the surface membrane of normal T lymphocytes, malignant T cells, and some malignant B cells such as CLL cells. The objective of this study was to evaluate the clinical response, the optimal dose and toxicity, and the host immune response to multiple-dose administration of the T101 monoclonal antibody.

II. MATERIALS AND METHODS

A. Patient Eligibility

Adult patients with a histologically confirmed diagnosis of CLL or CTCL refractory to standard therapy were candidates for this study. The patient's malignant cells must have demonstrated reactivity with the T101 antibody ($>$50% above background staining). Patients must not have had cytotoxic chemotherapy, radiation therapy, or immunosuppressant drugs for four weeks prior to entry into this trial. Patients must have had normal renal and hepatic function and no serious unrelated diseases. Patients must have been fully ambulatory with a Karnofsky performance status of $>$70% and a life expectancy of $>$2 months.

B. Study Plan

Six patients were to be entered at each fixed dose level (1,10,50,100, and 500mg): three patients with B cell disease and three patients with T cell disease. Patients were treated twice weekly for four weeks. If a response was demonstrated, they could continue at the same dosage. If no response was documented and there was no grade III or IV toxicity, they could be reentered at a higher dose level. Patients initially received T101 antibody through a peripheral vein in 100cc normal saline with 5% human albumin over two hours. This was later amended so that no more than 1-2mg of T101 antibody was infused per hour. Patients were carefully monitored for clinical response and toxicity, levels of circulating tumor antigen, antigen-antibody complexes, free antibody, antigenic modulation of tumor cells, and anti-murine antibody formation.

C. Toxicology of T101 Monoclonal Antibody

The T101 murine-derived monoclonal antibody was produced from ascites fluid and tested for endotoxin and contamination as previously described (10). The final concentration of immunoglobulin was measured by radioimmunodiffusion against a standard anti-mouse IgG_{2a} and was greater than 80% pure IgG_{2a}. The T101 antibody with an approved Investigational New Drug (IND) application with the Office of Biologics of the U.S. Food and Drug Administration was the generous gift of Hybritech, Inc., San Diego, California, under a collaborative study arrangement.

D. Surface Marker Analysis

Peripheral blood lymphocytes were isolated on a Ficoll-Hypaque density gradient. When monoclonal antibodies were tested in vitro they were used at a concentration of 1.25 to 2.5μg of antibody protein per $1x10^6$ cells. FITC-conjugated goat anti-mouse IgG secondary antibody was obtained from Tago, Inc. (Burlingame, CA). Purified mouse IgG_{2a} myeloma protein was used as a negative control (RPC-5, Bethesda Research Laboratories, Rockville, MD). Preparation of cells for immunofluorescence has previously been described (17). Flow cytometry analysis was performed on a 50H Cytofluoragraf (Ortho Diagnostic Systems, Inc., Westwood, MA). In vivo binding of T101 antibody was detected by incubation of cell suspensions directly with the FITC-conjugated goat anti-mouse IgG secondary antibody in vitro. Relative antigen density was determined by comparison of the mean fluorescence intensity over a 1,000 channel scale between specimens prepared and stained under identical conditions on the same day.

III. RESULTS

A. Chronic Lymphocytic Leukemia

Ten patients with CLL were entered into this protocol, and eight have completed the study (Table 1). The first patient was entered at 1mg and had no demonstrable change in peripheral blood counts following therapy despite the fact that cells were labeled in vivo with T101. Two other patients treated with 1mg demonstrated a transient 50% reduction in circulating CLL cells immediately following therapy that rose back to the baseline over the next six to twelve hours.

Three CLL patients were entered at the 10mg dose, and all three completed the full four weeks of therapy (eight doses). Two of them demonstrated a 50% reduction of their circulating leukemia cells that was sustained during the four weeks of therapy. Because of the peripheral blood response, one of these two patients continued at the 10mg dose for an additional four weeks; while CLL counts remained reduced, there was no reduction in the size of lymph nodes or organs. Interestingly, the T65 antigen on the leukemic cells underwent a decrease in density following the initial dose, and remained reduced throughout the course of therapy (Figure 1). While on T101 therapy at a 10mg dose, one of these three patients had progression of circulating leukemia cells, lymph nodes, and organs.

Bone marrow cells were studied prior to therapy and immediately following a 10mg dose. In vivo labeling with T101 was demonstrated following infusion with T101, as was reduction of the T65 antigen (Figures 2a and 2b). Not all of the antigenic sites were saturated in vivo, as increased staining was demonstrated when additional T101 was added. A lymph node was removed five hours following the infusion of 10mg of T101 into this same patient, and in vivo staining could not be demonstrated.

Four CLL patients were entered at the 50mg dose. Two were removed from study because of pulmonary toxicity. The other two patients are currently being treated with 50-hour infusions (1mg/hour) without major complications. It is still too early in their course to determine whether they will have a beneficial response; however, all of these patients developed a 50% reduction in circulating CLL cells immediately following each course of therapy. Bone marrow cells demonstrated minimal in vivo labeling which appeared to be related to extreme modulation of the T65 antigen. No in vivo labeling of lymph node cells could be identified following a 50-hour infusion of 50mg of T101.

TABLE 1. T101 Monoclonal Antibody Therapy of Chronic Lymphocytic Leukemia

Patient	Rai stage	Dose of T101 (mg)	Lymphocyte count		Nodes	Organs	Toxicity
			Pre-study	Post-study			
KK	IV	1 (8 doses)	23,000	41,000	stable	stable	urticaria, pulmonary
		50 (1 dose)					(50 mg)
AT	IV	1 (8 doses)	59,000	66,000	stable	stable	none
LK	IV	1 (6 doses)	56,000	46,000	stable	stable	none
HH	IV	10 (8 doses)	34,000	18,000	stable	stable	urticaria, fever
LM	IV	10 (16 doses)	5,000	3,000	stable	enlarged	urticaria, fever
AW	IV	10 (8 doses)	95,000	214,000	enlarged	enlarged	fever
AR	IV	50 (1 dose)	–	–	–	–	pulmonary
AO	IV	50 (3 doses)	–	–	–	–	urticaria, pulmonary fever
IF	IV	50 (6 doses)	290,000	290,000	stable	stable	urticaria, fever
AV	IV	50 (8 doses)	–	–	stable	stable	fever

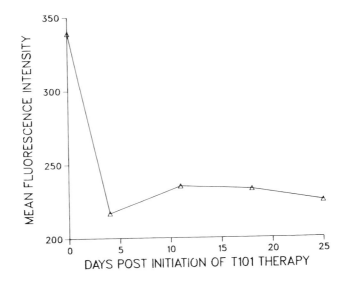

FIGURE 1.   Flow cytometry demonstrated a decrease in
expression of the T101 antigen throughout the four weeks of
therapy.   Each measurement was performed just prior to the
next dose when antigen expression should be maximal.   A
decrease or modulation of antigen expression is represented by
a decrease in mean fluorescence intensity.

B.   Cutaneous T-Cell Lymphoma

Seven patients with CTCL have been entered on this trial
(Table 2).   Two patients were treated at the 1mg dose level.
Neither of these patients demonstrated a clinical response to

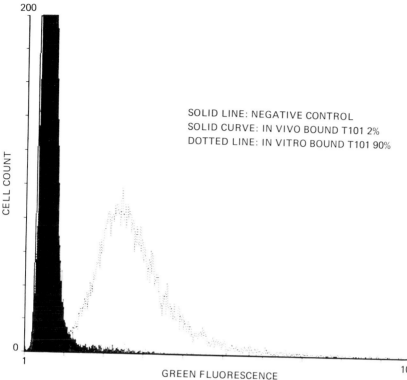

FIGURE 2a.   Binding of T101 antibody by bone marrow cells
prior to therapy.   The solid line represents the negative
control (FITC–conjugated RPC–5).   The solid curve represents
the in vivo bound T101, which parallels the control curve as
would be expected prior to T101 therapy.   The dotted line
represents in vitro bound T101 following incubation with
excess antibody.

T101 at 1mg.   Both of these patients were also treated at the
10mg dose.   One had improvement in skin lesions and a 50%
reduction in circulating cells on 10mg, but no change in lymph
nodes, hypercalcemia, or abnormal liver enzymes.   The other

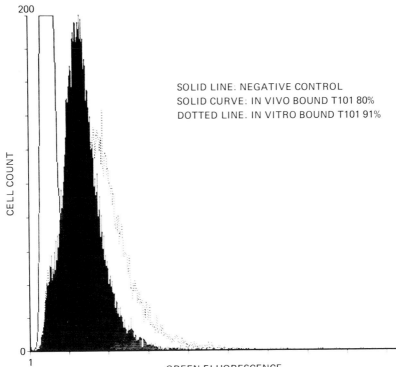

FIGURE 2b. Binding of T101 antibody by bone marrow cells two hours after T101 infusion. The solid line represents the negative control (FITC-conjugated RPC-5). The solid curve represents the in vivo bound T101, while the dotted line represents the sum of both in vivo and in vitro bound T101. The difference between the latter curves at two hours post infusion (11%) represents those bone marrow cells not saturated by T101 in vivo. The shift of the in vitro curve to the left indicates decreased intensity of staining of the leukemia cells probably due to antigenic modulation.

patient had no demonstrable change in skin lesions. Three patients were entered at the 10mg dose level and two of them were increased to the 50mg level after four weeks of treatment. There was gradual improvement in the skin lesions in all three of these patients.[2] There was no demonstrable response in lymph nodes or visceral metastases, however.

TABLE 2. T101 Monoclonal Antibody Therapy of Cutaneous T-Cell Lymphoma

Patient	CTCL stage	Dose of T101 (mg)	Type of skin lesions	Skin lesions	Organs	Nodes	Circulating Sézary cells	Toxicity
HB	IIB	1 (8 doses) 10 (8 doses)	tumors	stable	-	-	-	None
OB	IVB	1 (2 doses) 10 (2 doses) 50 (8 doses)	tumors	improved	stable	stable	probable decrease	None
WF	IVB	10 (on study)	generalized erythema	improved	stable	stable	-	pulmonary, fever
RB	IVA	10 (8 doses) 50 (7 doses)	generalized plaques	improved	-	stable	stable	pulmonary, fever
MM	IVB	10 (8 doses) 50 (8 doses)	generalized erythema and tumors	improved	stable	stable	stable	back pain and malaise, fever
JS	III	50 (3 doses)	generalized erythema	stable	-	-	stable	pulmonary, fever
ME	IVA	50 (8 doses) 100 (on study)	tumors	stable	-	-	-	pulmonary, fever

Skin biopsies were performed from 2–24 hours after the infusion of T101 antibody and studied for in vivo labeling of T101 by immunoperoxidase. Five patients had a total of 19 skin biopsies following T101 infusion. Eight biopsy specimens from four patients demonstrated in vivo localization of T101 (Figure 3).[2] Most of these were 2–24 hours following 50mg dosages; however, weak staining was identified in two biopsies after 10mg infusions of T101. Most of the in vivo localization was in the upper dermis. In a number of specimens, significant modulation of the T65 antigen was apparent (excess T101 was added in vitro and there was markedly reduced staining compared to pretreatment staining of skin lesions with T101, while the intensity of staining with the anti–Leu–4 antibody remained unchanged). In one patient a Pautrier's abscess demonstrated intense in vivo labeling with T101.

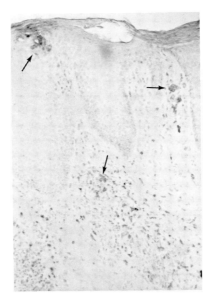

FIGURE 3. In vivo labeling of a mycosis skin lesion two hours after a 50mg dosage of T101 (arrows point to positive cells). Speciments were frozen in liquid nitrogen and stained with goat anti–mouse by the peroxidase anti–peroxidase technique. Additional T101 was not added in vitro.

---

[2]This information was not available on January 13, 1983, when this work was presented at the Armand Hammer Cancer Symposium.

C. Toxicity

Approximately 50% of the patients treated at the 10mg and 50mg dose levels developed urticaria. This could always be controlled with antihistamines and could often be prevented during subsequent infusions with T101 by pretreatment with antihistamines. Most patients developed fevers ranging from 99°F to 102°F during the infusion of T101. These were generally mild and rapidly relieved by acetaminophen. Three CLL patients treated with 50mg of T101, two of the CTCL patients treated with 50mg of T101, and one CTCL patient treated with 10mg of T101 developed shortness of breath and chest tightness during therapy. In all cases except one, no further therapy was given. Some patients developed this toxicity during their first infusion of T101, while one patient developed it during the eighth course of 50mg of T101. One patient developed a small pulmonary infiltrate coincident with this pulmonary toxicity that resolved over the next two weeks. Another patient developed a lung scan abnormality without a change in arterial blood gases following an episode of shortness of breath. The lung scan abnormality resolved two days later. We were unable to demonstrate an IgE anti-murine response using a sensitive enzyme-linked immunosorbent assay (ELISA) in patients who developed this pulmonary side effect. Skin tests were performed (0.01-0.00001 ng) in a number of patients; most of them demonstrated erythema within 20 minutes, but this did not correlate with systemic side effects. It was our opinion that this toxicity was most likely secondary to leukoagglutination leading to emboli in the microcirculation of the lungs. We therefore slowed the infusion rate to 1-2mg/hour. One patient who developed shortness of breath during a two-hour infusion of 10mg had no further problems when 10mg were infused over ten hours. Two other patients with CLL treated with 50mg infusions over 50 hours have had no problems during their therapy.

IV. DISCUSSION

We have demonstrated that at a 1mg or greater dose of T101, circulating CLL cells were stained with antibody and there was a rapid reduction in circulating CLL cells. In some patients this was maintained over the course of therapy. Partial antigenic modulation was demonstrated to persist throughout the course of T101 therapy in some patients. T101 at the 10mg and 50mg dose was demonstrated to bind in vivo and cause a transient modulation of the T101 antigen on bone marrow cells. We did not detect in vivo binding of T101 to lymph node cells or antigenic modulation five hours following a 10mg dose.

Seven patients with CTCL have been treated at 1, 10 and 50mg doses and four have demonstrated a response to this therapy with improvement in their skin lesions. T101 antibody was demonstrated to bind in vivo to the skin lesions in all four of these patients. Most of the staining was in the upper dermis, and antigenic modulation of the T65 antigen could be demonstrated in two of these patients.

The potentially serious side effect of shortness of breath and chest tightness was demonstrated in three CLL patients treated at the 50mg dose. This side effect resolved in minutes to a few hours and no residual effects were apparent. This reaction was sometimes associated with urticaria and was not prevented by pretreatment with hydroxyzine and cimetidine. We did not witness this side effect when the infusion was slowed to 1mg/hour in two CLL patients treated with 50mg of T101. Two patients with CTCL treated with 50mg of T101 and one at 10mg have also demonstrated pulmonary toxicity similar to that described in CLL patients. The T101 was being given at a rate of 10mg/hour. One patient demonstrated a transient infiltrate on chest X-ray and another patient demonstrated an abnormality on lung scan coincident with this side effect.

These data suggest that this pulmonary toxicity may be related to leukoagglutination secondary to relatively rapid infusion of T101 into patients who have circulating cells expressing the T65 antigen. One patient who developed this side effect following a two-hour infusion of 10mg had no problems following ten-hour infusions of 10mg (seven infusions total).

We are currently treating all of our patients at an infusion rate of 1-2mg/hour and, after twenty treatments in four different patients (two CLL, two CTCL), have not witnessed this side effect. At the end of a 50-hour infusion, however, bone marrow and circulating leukemia cells demonstrated little in vivo labeling, and additional T101 added in vitro demonstrated extreme modulation of the T65 antigen. These data suggest that while this prolonged infusion of T101 may prevent the pulmonary toxicity witnessed at more rapid infusions, antigenic modulation associated with this prolonged toxicity may render this therapy ineffective.

ACKNOWLEDGMENTS

We would like to thank Hybritech for kindly providing T101 antibody, Drs. Ivor Royston, Robert Dillman, and Dennis Carlo for their consultation and helpful suggestions, and the physicians and nurses of the Biological Response Modifiers Program and the Clinical Oncology Program for their invaluable help in carrying out this study. We would also like to thank Dr. Dean Metcalfe for performing the IgE anti-murine antibody ELISA, Richard Klein for technical assistance, Dr. Annette Maluish for assistance in specimen processing, and Dr. Adi Gazdar for photographing the skin biopsies presented in this manuscript.

ABBREVIATIONS

CLL, chronic lymphocytic leukemia; CTCL, cutaneous T cell lymphoma; ELISA, enzyme-linked immunosorbent assay.

REFERENCES

1. Rosenberg, S.A. and Terry, W.D. Adv. Cancer Res. 25, 323 (1977).
2. Wright, P.W., Hellstrom, I., and Bernstein, I.D. Med. Clin. North Am. 60, 607 (1976).
3. Fisher, R.I., Silver, B.A., Van Haelen, C.P., Jaffe, E.S., and Cossman, J. Cancer Res. 42, 2465 (1982).
4. Nadler, L.M., Stashenko, P., Hardy, R., Kufe, D.W., Antman, K.H. and Schlossm, S.R. Cancer Res. 40, 3147 (1980).
5. Miller, R.A., Maloney, D.G., McKillop, J., and Levy, R., Blood 58, 78 (1981).
6. Ritz, J., Pesando, J.M., Sallan, S.E., Clavell, L.A., Motismoc, J., Rosenthal, P. and Schlossm, S.F. Blood 58, 141 (1981).
7. Miller, R.A. and Levy, R. Lancet, August 1, 226 (1981).
8. Ritz, J. and Schlossman, S. Blood 59, 1 (1982).
9. Miller, R.A., Maloney, E.G., Warnke, R., and Levy, R. New Eng. J. Med. 306, 517 (1982).

10. Dillman, R.O., Shawler, D.L., Sobol, R.E., Shawler, D. L., Sobol, R.E., Collins, H.A., Beaurega, J.C., Wormsley, S.B. and Royston, I. Blood 59, 1036 (1982).

11. Sobol, R.E., Dillman, R.O., Smith, J.D., Imai, K., Ferrone, S., Shawler, D., Glassy, M.C. and Royston, I. in 'Progress in Cancer Research and Therapy' (M.S. Mitchell and H.F. Oettgen, eds.), Vol. 21, p. 199. Raven Press, New York (1982).

12. Sears, H.F., Mattis, J., Herlyn, D., Hayry, P., Atkinson, B., Ernst, C., Steplews, Z. and Koproski, H. Lancet, April 3, 762 (1982).

13. Foon, K.A., Schroff, R.W., and Gale, R.P. Blood 60, 1 (1982).

14. Foon, K.A., Bernhard, M.I., and Oldham, R.K. J. Biol. Resp. Modif. 1(3), 277 (1982).

15. Oldham, R.K., in 'Biological Response Modifiers in Human Oncology and Immunology' (H. Friedman, T. Klein and S. Spector, eds.) Plenum Press, New York (in press).

16. Royston, I., Majda, J.A., Baud, S.M., Meserve, B.L., and Griffiths, J.C. J. Immunol. 125, 725 (1980).

17. Schroff, R.W., Foon, K.A., Billing, R.J., and Fahey, J.L. Blood 59, 207 (1982).

THERAPEUTIC POTENTIAL OF MONOCLONAL ANTIBODIES THAT BLOCK BIOLOGICAL FUNCTION[1]

Ian S. Trowbridge

Cancer Biology Laboratory
The Salk Institute for Biological Studies
La Jolla, California

I. INTRODUCTION

The potential therapeutic uses of monoclonal antibodies in the treatment of cancer have attracted considerable interest in the last few years. Attention has mainly been focused upon two approaches: serotherapy, which relies upon the host immunological effector mechanisms to eliminate antibody-coated tumor cells, and the so-called magic bullet approach which involves selectively targeting covalently-bound drugs or toxins to the malignant tissue. The current status of this work is reviewed elsewhere in this volume (see, for example, the articles by Levy, Uhr and Thorpe). Here I wish to consider the advantages and limitations of a third general approach to cancer therapy employing monoclonal antibodies that act as pharmacological agents to directly block biological functions essential for cell proliferation. This is exemplified by the studies I will describe with monoclonal antibodies against the transferrin receptor.

---

[1]This work was supported by Grant CA34787 from the National Cancer Institute and funds donated by the Armand Hammer Foundation, the Paul Stock Foundation, the Helen K. and Arthur E. Johnson Foundation, BankAmerica Foundation, Mr. and Mrs. Lyndon C. Whitaker Charitable Foundation, Frances and Charles G. Haynsworth and Constance and Edward L. Grund.

Transferrin receptors facilitate the uptake of iron by binding Fe-transferrin and mediating its transport across the plasma membrane. In addition to being expressed in large quantities on normal tissues with high requirements for iron, such as maturing erythroid cells and placenta, transferrin receptors are found in abundance on proliferating cells from other tissues (1-5). As a consequence of their association with cell proliferation, as most clearly documented by a recent immunohistological study of normal human tissue and tumor biopsies using anti-transferrin receptor antibodies by David Mason and his colleagues (6), transferrin receptors are selectively expressed on a variety of tumors relative to most normal tissues (6-8).

II. RESULTS AND DISCUSSION

Although most monoclonal antibodies against the human transferrin receptor such as B3/25 (4), T56/14 (4), 5E9 (9) and OKT9 (5,10) do not interfere significantly with receptor function, by the appropriate screening procedures we were able to obtain a mouse anti-human receptor monoclonal antibody, designated 42/6, that blocks the binding of transferrin (11). As previously described, this antibody had a profound effect upon the growth of a human T leukemic cell line, CCRF-CEM, in vitro. A rat monoclonal antibody against the mouse transferrin receptor has also been obtained that blocks receptor function and inhibits in vitro growth of some tumor cell lines (12). As shown in Figure 1, both antibodies specifically interfere with transferrin-mediated iron uptake in cells of the appropriate species. With each monoclonal antibody the degree of inhibition of iron uptake from transferrin varies from 50% to greater than 90% depending upon the cell line tested. This variability in the inhibitory effects of the anti-transferrin receptor monoclonal antibodies on different cells together with differences in the absolute rates of iron uptake by particular cell types may have important implications for the possible clinical use of anti-transferrin receptor antibodies in cancer, as discussed later.

Because a rat monoclonal antibody is available that blocks transferrin receptor function in mice, it has been possible to test the in vivo antitumor activity of an anti-transferrin receptor antibody that blocks iron uptake into cells in a mouse model system. For our initial experiments, we chose the transplantable AKR mouse T cell leukemia, SL-2.

This is the cell line previously used by Bernstein and his colleagues to investigate the requirements for effective serotherapy with anti-Thy1 monoclonal antibodies (13,14). These earlier studies provide us with a standard against which to compare the antitumor activity of anti-transferrin receptor antibodies. This model is also attractive in that, if therapeutic effects are obtained with the transplantable T cell leukemia, studies can then be extended to include spontaneous T cell leukemias in AKR mice. Furthermore, it is known that T cell leukemias in man frequently express high numbers of transferrin receptors (4,5,10,15) and the in vitro growth of human T leukemic cell lines is particularly sensitive to the effects of monoclonal antibody 42/6 (11). Consequently, T cell leukemias might be expected to be a favorable starting point for attempting immunotherapy with anti-transferrin receptor antibodies.

We have now completed several trials of immunotherapy with the purified anti-mouse transferrin receptor antibody RI7 208 using the SL-2 leukemia model. The results have been quite encouraging. First, intravenous or interperitoneal injection of the monoclonal antibody had a significant effect upon the growth of SL-2 cells inoculated at a subcutaneous site. This was manifested not only as prolonged survival of tumor-bearing mice but also in marked inhibition of growth of the tumor at the primary site (Figure 2). This latter observation is in contrast to the relative ineffectiveness of the anti-Thy1 antibody, 19E12, used by Bernstein to inhibit growth of the primary subcutaneous site (13,14). An early example of such an experiment is shown in Figures 2 and 3. In this case, only two injections of RI7 208 monoclonal antibody were given, yet the antitumor effects of the immunotherapy are evident. Whereas untreated mice had a mean survival time of 23.8 ± 1.9 days, mice given 3mg of antibody i.v. on day 0 and 2mg of antibody i.p. on day 5 survived 31.3 ± 1.2 days. In subsequent trials, more prolonged treatments have proven to be even more effective. It should be noted that another rat monoclonal antibody against the mouse transferrin receptor, RI7 217, which does not inhibit receptor function (16, J. Lesley and R. Schulte, unpublished results) had little effect on tumor growth or host survival, consistent with the notion that RI7 208 monoclonal antibody is affecting cell growth in vivo by interfering with iron uptake.

The other major point of importance concerning the in vivo administration of the rat anti-mouse transferrin receptor monoclonal antibody RI7 208, in view of the fact that transferrin receptors are expressed on proliferating normal cells, is that so far there has been no evidence of

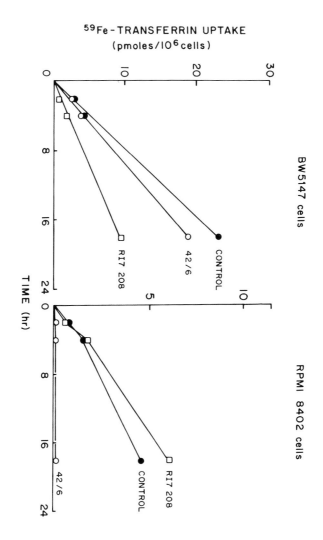

⁵⁹Fe-TRANSFERRIN UPTAKE
(pmoles/10⁶ cells)

BW5147 cells

RPMI 8402 cells

TIME (hr)

RI7 208

42/6

CONTROL

acute toxicity in the treated mice. It is not yet clear what the long-term effects of in vivo administrtion of the anti-body on normal tissues might be. However, there is good evidence that the pluripotent hemotopoietic stem cells (CFU-S) in adult mouse bone marrow do not express detectable numbers of transferrin receptors (D.L. Domingo and I.S. Trowbridge, unpublished results), and there are many possible reasons why some tumors may prove to be much more sensitive to the effects of anti-transferrin receptor antibodies that block iron uptake than most normal tissues. These include elevated levels of transferrin receptors on particular tumors relative to normal dividing cells, minor changes in receptor structure that affect antibody binding such as abnormal glycosylation that may occur in some malignant cells, as well as the accessibility of antibodies to the tumor mass relative to normal tissues. Another real possibility, for which evidence already exists (12), is that selective antitumor activity may be obtained because the consequences of iron deprivation for different cell types may vary. In other words, inhibiting the iron uptake of some cells by 90% may be rapidly lethal, yet other kinds of cells may, for a variety of reasons, tolerate deprivation of exogenous iron for much longer periods of time. Thus, the extent to which selec-tivity for tumor cells can be achieved in vivo with mono-clonal antibodies against functional cell surface receptors is difficult to predict a priori and will have to be

FIGURE 1. Inhibition of Transferrin-mediated Fe Uptake by Monoclonal Antibodies Against Human and Murine Transferrin Receptors. ^{59}Fe-human transferrin (specific activity 8.7×10^3 cpm per μg) was prepared as described previously (12) using the nitrilotriacetic acid method. Hematopoietic tumor cell lines were incubated at a cell density of 5×10^6 per ml in serum-free Dulbecco's modified Eagles medium containing 25μg/ml of ^{59}Fe-transferrin. Cell samples were removed at various times, washed in 0.15 M NaCl, 0.01 M Na phosphate buffer pH 7.2 containing 0.1% bovine serum albumin and counted in a gamma counter. Cells treated with purified monoclonal antibody were incubated with 50μg/ml antibody for 30 minutes at 37°C prior to the addition of labeled trans-ferrin. In all experiments, radioactivity associated with cells harvested immediately after addition of ^{59}Fe-transferrin was determined and subtracted from values of Fe uptake. BW5147 is a mouse T lymphoma cell line and RPMI 8402 is a human T cell lymphoma cell line.

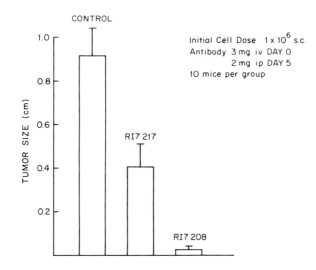

FIGURE 2. Rat Anti-murine Transferrin Receptor Monoclonal Antibody, RI7 208, Inhibits the Growth of SL-2 Leukemic Cells at the Primary Tumor Site. The figure shows the mean tumor size (measured as the average of two perpendicular axes with calipers) of groups of mice ten days after inoculation of 1×10^6 SL-2 cells at a subcutaneous site on the lower back. RI7 217 is a rat anti-murine transferrin receptor monoclonal antibody that does not block receptor function.

determined for individual monoclonal antibodies directed against each receptor. In view of other problems associated with serotherapy and drug targeting, such as heterogeneity of antigen expression on tumors and antigenic modulation that may be less severe in the case of functional receptors (17), the idea of using monoclonal antibodies to block the function of essential growth-related receptors seems worth further investigation. Monoclonal antibodies have been obtained against the epidermal growth factor receptor (18), the insulin receptor (19,20) and the interleukin 2 (IL-2)

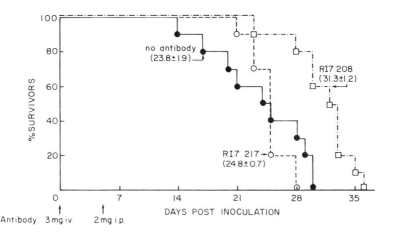

FIGURE 3. Treatment of AKR Mice with Rat Anti-murine Transferrin Receptor Antibody, RI7 208, Prolongs Survival of Mice Challenged with SL-2 Leukemia Cells. The data are from the same experiment shown in Figure 2 in which mice were inoculated with 1×10^6 SL-2 cells at a subcutaneous site and then given monoclonal antibodies as described. The figures in parentheses are the mean survival times for each treatment group $\pm$ 1 std. error.

receptor of human cells (21). It has been shown that the monoclonal antibody designated TAC against the IL-2 receptor blocks IL-2 binding and inhibits the in vitro growth of human T lymphocytes (21). If tissue-specific growth-related receptors analogous to IL-2 receptors on T lymphocytes can be identified on epithelial cells, the prospects of using mono-clonal antibodies to treat the common carcinomas that constitute the major human cancers will be considerably brighter.

ABBREVIATIONS

IL-2, interleukin 2.

REFERENCES

1. Larrick, J.W. and Cresswell, P.   J. Supramol. Struct.
    11, 576 (1979).
2. Hamilton, T.A., Wada, H.G., and Sussman, H.H. Proc.
    Natl. Acad. Sci. USA 76, 6406 (1979).
3. Galbraith, G.M.P., Galbraith, R.M., and Faulk, W.P.
    Cell Immunol. 49, 215 (1980).
4. Trowbridge, I.S. and Omary, M.B., Proc. Natl. Acad. Sci.
    USA 78, 3039 (1981).
5. Sutherland, R., Delia, D., Schneider, C., Newman, R.,
    Kemshead, J., and Greaves, M. Proc. Natl. Acad. Sci.
    USA, 78, 4515 (1981).
6. Gatter, K.C., Brown, G., Trowbridge, I.S.,
    Woolston, R.E., and Mason, D.Y. J. Clin. Path., Vol.
    36, p. 539 (1983).
7. Faulk, W.P., Hsi, B-L., and Stevens, P.L. Lancet,
    August 23, 390 (1980).
8. Shindelman, J.E., Ortmeyer, A.E., and Sussman, H.H.
    Int. J. Cancer 27, 329 (1981).
9. Haynes, B.F., Hemler, M., Cotner, T., Mann, D.L.,
    Eisenbarth, G.S., Strominger, J.L., and Fauci, A.S. J.
    Immunol. 127, 347 (1981).
10. Reinherz, E.L., Kung, P.C., Goldstein, G., Levy, R.H.,
    and Schlossman, S.F. Proc. Natl. Acad. Sci. USA 77,
    1588 (1980).
11. Trowbridge, I.S. and Lopez, F. Proc. Natl. Acad. Sci.
    USA, 79, 1175 (1982).
12. Trowbridge, I.S., Lesley, J., and Schulte, R. J. Cell.
    Physiol. 112, 403 (1982).
13. Bernstein, I.D., Tam, M.R., and Nowinski, R.C. Science
    207, 68 (1980).
14. Bernstein, I.D. and Nowinski, R.C., in 'Hybridomas in
    Cancer Diagnosis and Treatment' (M.S. Mitchell and H.F.
    Oettgen, eds.), p. 97 Raven Press, New York (1982).
15. Omary, M.B., Trowbridge, I.S., and Minowada, J. Nature
    (London) 286, 888 (1980).
16. Trowbridge, I.S. and Domingo, D.L. Cancer Surveys 1,
    543 (1982).
17. Trowbridge, I.S. and Domingo, D.L. Nature 294, 171
    (1981).

18. Schreiber, A.B., Lax, I., Yarden, Y., Eshhar, Z., and Schlessinger, J. Proc. Natl. Acad. Sci. USA 78, 7535 (1981).

19. Kull, F.C., Jacobs, S., Su, Y-F., and Cuatrecasas, P. Biochem. Biophys. Res. Comm. 106, 1019 (1982).

20. Roth, R.A., Cassell, D.J., Wong, K.Y., Maddux, B.A., and Goldfine, I.D. Proc. Natl. Acad. Sci. USA 79, 7312 (1982).

21. Leonard, W.J., Depper, J.M., Uchiyama, T., Smith, K.A., Waldmann, T.A., and Greene, W.C. Nature 300, 267 (1982).

QUESTIONS AND ANSWERS

GUPTA: There is a widespread cytotoxic effect of monoclonal antibodies against transferrin receptors in vitro in contrast to a modest effect in vivo. What is the reason for this paradoxical effect?

TROWBRIDGE: The antibody arrests growth, and in vivo there are only 2-3 logs of cell killing.

KAPLAN: Have you looked at the SL-2 cells that survive, to see if there is any selection for cells with altered expression of the transferrin receptor?

TROWBRIDGE: Yes. As far as we can tell there is not any evidence for modulation.

TAYLOR-PAPADIMITRIOU: (Comment) Within the context of inhibiting tumor cell growth by interfering with the interaction of growth factors, it may be that a more specific antitumor effect could be obtained using antibodies to growth factors rather than to their receptors. The 'transforming factors' produced by many tumor cells could be important in tumor progression but not necessary for normal cell growth. Antibodies to such factors may, therefore, be suitable for in vivo inhibition of metastatic tumor cells.

PROSPECTS FOR ANTIBODY THERAPY OF LEUKEMIA:
EXPERIMENTAL STUDIES IN MURINE LEUKEMIA[1]

Christopher C. Badger
Irwin D. Bernstein

Medical Oncology and Pediatric Oncology Programs,
Fred Hutchinson Cancer Research Center; and
Departments of Medicine and Pediatrics,
University of Washington School of Medicine,
Seattle, Washington

I. INTRODUCTION

Monoclonal antibodies against cell surface differentiation antigens have been used to treat a variety of experimental and clinical tumors (1-14). Unfortunately, with the exception of anti-idiotypic antibody treatment of a B cell lymphoma (2), results of clinical trials have thus far been disappointing, possibly because patients with end stage disease and large tumor burdens have been treated. To better understand reasons for failure and to attempt to define more effective antibody regimens, a number of animal models have been developed. With these models it has been possible to inhibit the outgrowth of limited numbers of transplanted tumor cells bearing the appropriate target antigen (3-14) and gain insight into possibly effective approaches to antibody treatment in humans.
     To define the variables which influence antibody mediated antitumor effects, we have used monoclonal antibodies against a murine T cell differentiation antigen, Thy1.1, to treat mice with transplanted T cell leukemia. In initial studies we were able to demonstrate that anti-Thy1.1 antibody could prevent

[1]This work was supported by grants CA26386 and CA33477 from the National Cancer Institute.

the outgrowth of an otherwise lethal dose of syngeneic
T leukemic cells without apparent adverse effects on the
host (9-14). Moreover, antibody of the IgG2a isotype was more
effective than antibody of the IgG3 isotype, and IgM was
ineffective when given in equal milligram doses (10). The
lack of effect of IgM antibody infusion, as well as the fact
that these studies were evaluated in C'5 deficient AKR/J mice
suggested that antibody acted by a cell-dependent rather than
complement-dependent mechanism.

In the following studies examining the therapeutic
potential of monoclonal antibodies against normal
differentiation antigens, we have utilized an IgG2a monoclonal
anti-Thy1.1 antibody 19E12, to successfully treat transplanted
syngeneic AKR/J SL2 T leukemic cells. Moreover, we have been
able to extend this approach to the treatment of spontaneously
occurring T cell leukemias in aged AKR/J mice. Below we first
briefly review our recent studies with transplanted leukemias.
Following, our preliminary attempts to treat naturally
occurring leukemia in mice are discussed. Details of these
tumor systems and the monoclonal antibody 19E12 have been
previously described (10,11).

II. ANTIBODY TREATMENT OF TRANSPLANTED LEUKEMIA

In a series of experiments we have examined dose-response
relationships, the maximal antileukemic effect of antibody and
the factors leading to the failure of antibody therapy in
transplanted leukemia (see reference 14 for details of studies
reviewed in this section).

A.   Dose-Response Relationships

The optimal single dose of antibody was determined by
treating mice implanted with $3x10^5$ cells with a single
intravenous infusion of ascites containing doses of 0.4 to
6.4mg of antibody. A dose of 3.2mg was most effective,
completely inhibiting tumor growth in 83% of the animals,
while lower doses (0.4mg or 1.2mg) cured a smaller percentage
of mice. Of interest, a higher dose of 6.4mg was also less
effective, curing only 22% of animals. To examine the
possibility that the decreased effectiveness of very high
doses of antibody was a result of the infusion of toxic
impurities in the large amounts of ascites fluid, a subsequent
experiment was performed using antibody purified by adsorption

and elution from staphlococcal protein A. In this study a dose of 1.5mg was the most effective, curing 80% of animals, and cure rates again decreased with higher doses. Thus, the decreased effectiveness of very high doses was due to the antibody itself rather than impurities in the ascites. This decrease in effectiveness may possibly have been a result of inhibition of effector cell function by very high levels of free antibody.

The ability of a single dose of antibody to eliminate leukemic cells was limited. When the inoculum was increased to $3x10^6$ cells, antibody in doses of 0.4–6.4mg of ascites or 0.5–16mg of purified antibody failed to cure any of the treated animals. Antibody therapy did, however, prolong survival in these animals, primarily by delaying the development of metastatic disease.

The possibility that prolonged therapy, by maintaining antibody levels and thus allowing more time for effector cells to localize to the site of tumor growth, would be more effective than a single dose was also evaluated. Animals were implanted with $3x10^5$ or $3x10^6$ cells and then treated with one of three regimens: 1) 3.6mg single infusion, 2) 3.6mg followed by four doses of 1.8mg over two weeks or 3) 0.4mg followed by four doses of 0.2mg. A control group remained untreated. In animals implanted with $3x10^5$ cells, both high dose regimens cured 80% of the animals and were more effective than the low-dose prolonged regimen, which cured 20% of the mice. When the tumor inoculum was increased to $3x10^6$ cells, antibody again failed to cure any animals, although survival was prolonged by all the antibody regimens. Thus, a single, relatively high dose (3.2–3.6mg) of antibody produced the maximal antileukemic effect (i.e., elimination of $3x10^5$ subcutaneous cells) and there was no advantage in giving multiple doses.

The basis of the requirement for high doses of antibody to achieve maximal effectiveness was examined by studying antibody binding to leukemic cells in vivo. Coating of leukemic cells by infused antibody was determined in animals bearing established subcutaneous tumor nodules. The amount of antibody bound to the cell surfaces was found to be directly related to the infused dosage of antibody, with doses of ≥ 3.2mg completely saturating cell surface antigenic sites. The most effective antileukemic dose, therefore, appeared to be the lowest dose capable of achieving maximal saturation of leukemic cell surfaces.

B.   Causes of Failure

When animals were implanted with 3×10^6 SL2 leukemic cells, antibody prolonged survival but failed to cure any animals. The failure to completely inhibit the growth of leukemia could have resulted from alterations in antigenic expression by the leukemic cells or from limitations in the ability of host effector mechanisms to eliminate antibody-coated cells. To evaluate these possibilities, Thy1.1 expression and the presence of infused anti-Thy1.1 antibody on the leukemic cell surfaces were determined on cells from subcutaneous nodules and on metastatic cells in the spleen, which had grown in spite of high-dose prolonged antibody therapy (3.6mg followed by 1.8mg x four doses) (14). Cells from the subcutaneous nodule maintained Thy1.1 expression in levels comparable to untreated controls and, furthermore, had near-maximal saturation of cell surface sites by the infused antibody.

In contrast, cells from the spleen were not coated with antibody and did not express Thy1.1. In additional studies, even low doses (0.4mg) of antibody resulted in antigen-negative metastases. These antigen-negative cells were shown to be stable variants since they maintained their antigen-negative phenotype following several in vivo passages in the absence of antibody.

Thus, the growth of a subcutaneous nodule resulted from the inability of the host to eliminate antibody-coated cells, while metastatic disease resulted from the emergence of antigen-negative variants. The prolonged survival noted following even low doses of antibody was presumably a result of the time necessary for the selection of these variants and suggested antibody was more efficient in eliminating circulating leukemic cells than in inhibiting subcutaneous growth. This may have been a result of effector cells having better access to the circulating leukemic cells.

III.   ANTIBODY TREATMENT OF SPONTANEOUS LEUKEMIA

The occurrence of spontaneous T cell leukemias in aged AKR/J mice provides a model more closely analogous to clinical leukemia than transplanted disease. We have, therefore, used antibody to treat aged AKR/J mice with spontaneous leukemia following remission induction with chemotherapy. Animals were treated in remission because, in preliminary experiments, antibody infusion in frankly leukemic mice led to rapid death from cell lysis and agglutination. In these studies, mice in our retired breeder colony were examined weekly and those developing leukemia were diagnosed clinically by enlargement of thymus, spleen or lymph nodes (15). These mice were treated with cyclophosphamide, 150mg/kg, i.p. on days 0 and 3 to induce a remission of the leukemia. Remission, as diagnosed by resolution of previously enlarged lymphoid organs, was achieved in 90% of mice by day 3. Animals in remission were randomized to receive or not receive antibody therapy. In a preliminary experiment, treatment with 19E12 antibody (0.4mg i.v. on day 3 followed by 0.2mg i.p. twice weekly until death) led to a significant, although modest, prolongation of relapse free survival (p = .01). In contrast to the results with transplanted leukemia, where animals uniformly died of leukemia or were long-term survivors, a number of antibody-treated animals died in remission. Thus, despite a significant prolongation of remission duration there was no difference in overall survival (11).

The improved relapse-free survival was confirmed in a subsequent experiment using the same antibody treatment regimen. An analysis of white blood cell counts (wbc) obtained prior to treatment revealed that the effect of antibody was primarily seen in animals with pretreatment wbcs of 10,000 to 20,000, where there was a doubling of median relapse-free survival. Furthermore, in this group there was a significant prolongation in absolute survival (p = .01) with a majority of antibody-treated animals dying in remission (12).

In a third experiment, we compared the prolonged antibody treatment described above to the regimen most effective in the treatment of transplanted tumors, a single dose of 3.2mg antibody, as well as to a single dose of 0.4mg on day 3. In addition, a control group in which mice were treated with ascites fluid containing a control IgG2a antibody of irrelevant specificity was also included. Thus, mice were treated with cyclophosphamide (150mg/kg, days 0 and 3), and those mice achieving remission were randomized into one of five treatments: 1) 19E12, 0.4mg day 3 then 0.2mg twice a week; 2) 19E12, 0.4mg day 3; 3) 19E12, 3.2mg day 3; 4) irrelevant antibody, 0.4mg day 3 then 0.2mg twice a week or 5) no further therapy. Comparison of mice treated versus not treated with 19E12 antibody revealed that treatment with antibody again resulted in a significant prolongation in relapse-free survival (p = .007) and remission duration (p < .001) but no improvement in overall survival (Figure 1). Analysis by treatment group showed no difference in survival or relapse-free survival among the three 19E12 regimens. There was no effect of the control antibody.

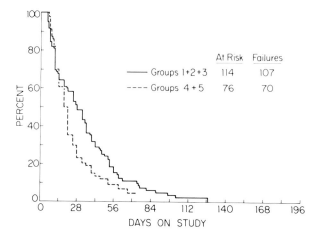

FIGURE 1.   Relapse-Free Survival: All Animals.   Aged
AKR/J mice with spontaneous leukemia were treated with
cyclophosphamide, 150mg/kg, i.p., days 0 and 3. Those animals
in remission on day 3 were randomized to antibody therapy:
Group 1) 19E12, 0.4mg i.v., day 3; Group 4) control antibody
of irrelevant specificity, 0.4mg i.v. day 3 followed by 0.2mg
i.p. twice weekly until death; Group 2) 19E12, 0.4mg i.v.
day 3; Group 3) 19E12, 3.2mg i.v. day 3; Group 4) control
antibody of irrelevant specificity, 0.4mg i.v. day 3 followed
by 0.2mg i.p. twice weekly until death; Group 5) no further
therapy. Time to relapse or death in remission is shown for
combined 19E12 treated groups and combined control groups.

When groups were stratified according to the pretreatment
wbc and the results in treated versus untreated groups were
compared, the influence of antibody treatment was seen again
predominantly in those animals with an intermediate wbc

(10–20,000) (Figure 2). For this group, antibody treatment resulted in a significant prolongation in survival (p = .033), relapse–free survival (p = .008) and time to relapse (p < .0001). There is not yet sufficient data to determine if one antibody regimen is superior in this subgroup.

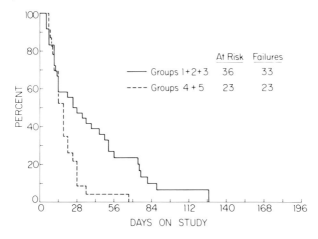

FIGURE 2. Relapse–Free Survival: WBC 10,000 to 20,000. AKR/J mice with spontaneous leukemia were treated as in Figure 1. Relapse–free survival of animals with pretreatment white blood counts between 10,000 and 20,000 is shown for combined 19E12 groups and combined control groups.

The reason that antibody treatment was most effective for mice with diagnostic wbc of 10–20,000 is not known. However, preliminary results from an ongoing experiment have suggested that the ineffectiveness of antibody therapy in animals with <10,000 wbc on diagnosis may have been a result of a high proportion of leukemias lacking Thy1.1 in these animals. In

animals with high (>20,000) wbc, failure of antibody therapy
may have resulted from a larger leukemic burden remaining
after chemotherapy or from decreased effector function, if wbc
reflected the degree of marrow infiltration by leukemic cells.

IV. TOXICITY OF ANTIBODY THERAPY

As noted earlier, in contrast to animals with transplanted
leukemia treated with antibody alone, a major proportion of
animals died in remission following therapy with
cyclophosphamide and 19E12 antibody. These nonleukemic deaths
occurred in two phases. Approximately 30–40% of animals died
between days 7 and 21. Death rates in this period were
similar for mice treated with 19E12 antibody and those treated
with cyclophosphamide alone or irrelevant antibody (see Figure
1). Histologic examination revealed that most of these
animals died of bacterial infection, primarily pneumonia,
pyelonephritis and extensive bacterial abscesses. This early
mortality was presumably due to myelosuppression from the
cyclophosphamide with subsequent bacterial infection.

After day 21 only 5% of control animals died prior to
clinical evidence of relapse. In contrast, 55% of
antibody-treated animals died between days 21 and 100 while in
clinical remission. Histologic examination revealed pneumonia
as the predominant cause of death in these animals. The late
nonleukemic mortality in antibody-treated animals may have
resulted from immunosuppression which occurred as a
consequence of treatment with cyclophosphamide and anti–T cell
antibody. In current studies we are attempting to prevent
these infections by increasing antibiotic support during
therapy.

V. DISCUSSION

Several principles of antibody therapy have begun to
emerge from these studies. In the case of extravascular
tumor, the ability of antibody alone to eliminate a
subcutaneous implant may be limited to a few hundred thousand
leukemic cells at a single site. High intravenous doses of
antibody were required to maximally coat tumor cells in the
subcutaneous space and produce consistent inhibition of an
implant of 3×10^5 cells. Larger numbers of subcutaneous cells

could not be eliminated, possibly because of a limitation of host effector mechanisms. In addition, we were unable to produce an increase in effectiveness by infusing multiple doses of antibody over time. These results suggest that when treating a rapidly growing extravascular tumor, antibody should be given over a short period of time in doses capable of saturating extravascular cell surfaces. Higher doses than those required to produce cell surface saturation may be less effective, although the reasons for this phenomenon are not known. Importantly, elimination of greater numbers of tumor cells in the extravascular space may require that antibody be used as a carrier for a cytotoxic agent so as to obviate the requirement for participation of host effector mechanisms.

In contrast, antibody can efficiently prevent metastatic spread of tumor cells. Relatively low doses of antibody that were incapable of eliminating extravascular tumor cells were able to prevent the spread of tumor cells which express the target antigen. Presumably, this was a result of more efficient removal of antibody-coated cells from the intravascular space. Thus, antibody may be useful in preventing dissemination of tumor cells, e.g., at surgery for primary tumor removal. The emergence of antigen-negative variants suggests that successful therapy may require multiple antibodies against multiple antigens to reduce the probability of such variants.

The antibody therapy of naturally occurring leukemias also shows promise. Our studies have shown that treatment with antibody during remission can induce a modest prolongation in disease-free survival. This effect was particularly dramatic in mice with wbc counts of 10-20,000 at diagnosis. The failure to achieve a clinically significant increase in survival was due to the high incidence of infection. Presumably, treatment with the combination of high doses of cyclophosphamide and anti-T cell antibody accounted for this high infection rate and institution of appropriate supportive care to prevent and treat infection should lead to marked improvement in the results of antibody treatment. Thus, provided that it is used in the clinic under appropriate conditions, such as those defined by the animal model, antibody against normal differentiation antigens may provide an effective antitumor reagent in the treatment of intravascular tumors, in particular leukemias and lymphomas.

ABBREVIATIONS

WBC, white blood cell count.

REFERENCES

1. Ritz, J. and Schlossman, S.F. Blood 59, 1 (1982).
2. Miller, R.A., Maloney, D.G., Warnke, R., and Levy, R. New
    Engl. J. Med. 306, 517 (1982).
3. Young, W.W., Jr. and Hakomori, S-I. Science 211, 487
    (1981).
4. Scheinberg, D.A. and Strand, M. Cancer Res. 42, 44
    (1982).
5. Kirch, M.E. and Hammerling, U. J. Immunol. 127, 805
    (1981).
6. Herlyn, D.M., Steplewski, Z., Herlyn, M.F., and
    Koprowski, H. Cancer Res. 40, 717 (1980).
7. Krolick, K.A., Uhr, J.W., Slavin, S., and Vitetta, E.S.
    J Exp. Med. 155, 1797 (1982).
8. Blythman, H.E., Casellas, P., Gros, O., Gros, P.,
    Jansen, F.K., Paolucci, F., Pau, B., and Vidal, H.
    Nature 290, 145 (1981).
9. Bernstein, I.D., Tam, M.R., and Nowinski, R.C. Science
    207, 68 (1980).
10. Bernstein, I.D., Nowinski, R.C., Tam, M.R., McMaster, B.,
    Houston, L.L., and Clark, E.A., in: 'Monoclonal
    Antibodies' (R.H. Kennett, T.J. McKearn, and
    K.B. Bechtol, eds.), p. 275, Plenum Publishing Corp., New
    York (1980).
11. Bernstein, I.D. and Nowinski, R.C., in: 'Hybridomas in
    Cancer Diagnosis and Treatment' (M.S. Mitchell and
    H.F. Oettgen, eds.), p. 97, Raven Press, New York (1982).
12. Badger, C.C. and Bernstein, I.D., in: 'Monoclonal
    Antibodies in Drug Development,' Proceedings of 1st John
    Jacob Abel Symposium on Drug Development (J.T. August,
    ed.), p. 151, American Society for Pharmacology and
    Experimental Therapeutics, Bethesda (1982).
13. Bernstein, I.D. and Badger, C.C., in: 'Rational Basis
    for Chemotherapy,' UCLA Symposia on Molecular and
    Cellular Biology, Vol. 1 (B.A. Chabner, ed.), Alan R.
    Liss, Inc., New York (in press).
14. Badger, C.C. and Bernstein, I.D. J. Exp. Med. (in
    press).
15. Kende, M., Goldberg, A.I., Glynn, J.P., Mantel, N., and
    Goldin, A. Cancer Chemother. Rep. 56, 683 (1972).

AUTOLOGOUS BONE MARROW TRANSPLANTATION FOR STAGE IV ABDOMINAL NON-HODGKIN'S LYMPHOMA AFTER IN VITRO PURGING WITH ANTI-Y 29/55 MONOCLONAL ANTIBODY AND COMPLEMENT

C. Baumgartner, P. Imbach, A. Luthy
and R. Odavic

Department of Pediatrics
University Hospitals, Inselspital
3010 Bern, Switzerland

H. P. Wagner

Department of Pediatrics
University Hospitals, Inselspital
3010 Bern, Switzerland
and
Institute for Clinical Experimental
Cancer Research, Tiefenauspital
3004 Bern, Switzerland

G. Brun del Re and U. Bucher

Central Hematology Laboratory
University Hospitals, Inselspital
3010 Bern, Switzerland

H. K. Forster

Central Research Units, F. Hoffmann-La Roche
and Co., Ltd., 4002 Basel, Switzerland

A. Hirt and A. Morell

Institute for Clinical and Experimental
Cancer Research, Tiefenauspital
3004 Bern, Switzerland

I. INTRODUCTION

Intensity of therapeutic regimens in advanced malignancies
is limited by severe toxicity to the hematopoietic system.
Experimental and clinical data demonstrate that the infusion
of autologous hematopoietic   stem cells can restore bone
marrow   function   after   application   of   supralethal
chemoradiotherapy (1,2).   Improved tumor control may be
expected from such procedures.   However, there is a
substantial risk that the reinfused remission marrow may
contain residual neoplastic cells.   In patients with acute
lymphoblastic leukemia, attempts have been made to eliminate
such residual blasts from the bone marrow by use of complement
and either heterologous antibodies (3) or monoclonal
antibodies (4).   Juvenile patients with stage IV abdominal
non-Hodgkin's lymphoma (NHL), particularly of the Burkitt's
type, have a poor prognosis (5).   For this reason, we
developed a protocol for such patients combining intensive
cytotoxic therapy and total body irradiation with autologous
bone marrow transplantation (ABMT) after in vitro purging of
the marrow using the B-leukemia-associated monoclonal antibody
anti-Y 29/55 (6) and complement.

II. MATERIALS, METHODS AND PATIENTS

A.   Cytoreductive Therapy

Patients received conventional induction therapy including
vincristine, adriamycin, cyclophosphamide and prednisone
together with intrathecal chemotherapy.   Cranial irradiation
was added if signs of central nervous system (CNS) involvement
were present.   High dose consolidation therapy with autologous
bone marrow rescue, as shown in Table 1, was performed as soon
as remission was achieved (2-3 months after diagnosis).
Systemic chemotherapy was discontinued therafter except for
intrathecal medication.

B.   Anti-Y 29/55

The monoclonal murine antibody anti-Y 29/55 (IgG2a,κ)
reacts with the malignant lymphocyte populations in peripheral
blood of patients with B cell chronic lymphocytic leukemia
(CLL), B-NHL, and hairy cell leukemia (6).   The antibody thus

TABLE 1. Pretransplant Regimen

Therapy	Day							
	−7	−6	−5	−4	−3	−2	−1	0
Vincristine 2mg/m^2 (max. 2mg) i.v.	V							
Adriamycin 60mg/m^2 i.v.	A							
Cyclophosphamide 45mg/kg i.v.		C	C	C	C			
Total body irradiation 600 rads							I	
Autologous bone marrow transplantation								T

recognizes neoplastic populations of human plasma cell
precursors, arrested at various stages of differentiation.
Anti-Y 29/55 binds also to non-malignant B lymphocytes
normally confined to secondary lymphoid organs such as lymph
nodes, spleen and tonsils. It does not react with malignant
cells of null acute lymphocytic leukemia (ALL), common ALL,
pre-B-ALL, T-ALL, T lymphoma, acute myeloid leukemia or
chronic myeloid leukemia.

C. Bone Marrow Processing

Optimal conditions for bone marrow treatment were
determined in a cytotoxicity assay using peripheral blood
cells of B-CLL patients. Approximately 80% of the target
cells were lysed at antibody concentrations above 0.1µl
ascites fluid per ml cell suspension (2x10^7 cells/ml)
(Figure 1). A similar proportion of cells were found to be
surface Ig positive. Based on these results, an at least
1000-fold excess of antibody was chosen for bone marrow
treatment. Growth of normal granulocyte-macrophage precursors
(CFU-c) was not significantly impaired by this procedure as
tested by the CFU-c assay performed before and after
cryopreservation (Figure 2). The bone marrow of the patients

was harvested after one or two courses of chemotherapy. At
this time the percentage of malignant cells was below 1%. The
mononuclear cell fraction was obtained by sodium
metrizoate/Ficoll density gradient centrifugation. Cells were
washed and resuspended in Hank's solution at a concentration
of $10-20 \times 10^6$/ml. The antibody (30–60µl ascites fluid per ml
cell suspension) and complement (rabbit serum, final
concentration 20%) were added and the suspension was incubated
for 90 minutes at 20^oc. Finally, the cells were washed twice
and cryopreserved as usual. No residual tumor cells were
detected after this procedure by indirect immunofluorescence
(2000 cells evaluated).

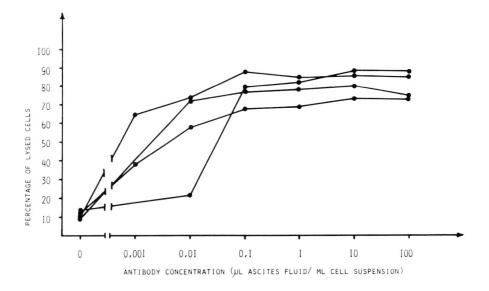

FIGURE 1. Incubation of CLL cells of four patients with
the antibody anti-Y 29/55 and complement: relation between
antibody concentration and cell lysis as shown by trypan blue
stain.

D. Patients

Three male patients (age 7, 10, and 14 years) have been
treated under this protocol. They all had histologically
proven disseminated malignant NHL (Burkitt's type) of

abdominal origin (the tumor cells reacted with anti-Y 29/55 as shown by indirect immunofluorescence). At presentation, bone marrow of all patients was infiltrated by the tumor. Two patients which had CNS involvement in addition received cranial irradiation before ABMT. In the post-transplant period, we observed complications like veno-occlusive disease of the liver in one patient (reversed within two months) and a severe polyneuropathy in another patient (slowly regressive). These were considered due to the cytoreductive therapy and not to the in vitro purging procedure of the bone marrow.

III. RESULTS

Hematopoietic recovery was observed in these patients, thus giving evidence of marrow engraftment. No delay was recorded, when compared to 16 ABMT patients with untreated marrow. The immunologic reconstitution was also similar in the two groups. In both cases we observed a predominance of suppressor T cells over helper T cells, a reversible deficit of B cells in the blood, and subnormal immunoglobulin levels in the first months following ABMT. The three stage IV NHL patients transplanted with in vitro-treated marrow are now surviving for 15+, 10+, and 8+ months in continued complete remission. In a previous study, ten patients with abdominal NHL of stage III and IV were treated under a similar regimen excluding bone marrow treatment. Tumor relapse occurred in all three patients with stage IV NHL and in two patients with stage III NHL. Relapses usually occurred within two to three months after ABMT, the latest being at six months.

IV. CONCLUSIONS

The monoclonal antibody anti-Y 29/55 effectively induces complement-mediated lysis of neoplastic B lymphoma cells without interfering with normal bone marrow elements. It can, therefore, be used to eradicate residual lymphoma cells from bone marrow prior to autologous transplantation.

Three high-risk patients with stage IV abdominal NHL of the Burkitt's type have received ABMT after in vitro bone marrow treatment. They all remain in complete remission 8+ to 15+ months after ABMT. Previous experience indicates recurrence of this tumor is unlikely if more than six months have passed after cessation of therapy. This suggests that

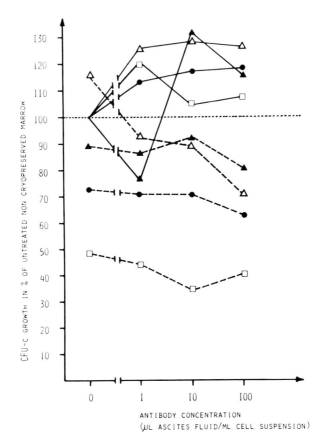

FIGURE 2.   CFU-c growth (before —— and after ---
cryopreservation) in bone marrow of 4 (Δ,▲,●,□)
hematologically normal donors after incubation with different
anti-Y 29/55 antibody concentrations and complement (cfu-c
growth of untreated noncryopreserved marrow = 100%).

our therapeutic regimen has been effective.   Further
experience, however, is required for final evaluation.

ABBREVIATIONS

NHL, non-Hodgkin's lymphoma; ABMT, autologous bone marrow
transplantation; CNS, central nervous system; CLL, chronic
lymphocytic leukemia; ALL, acute lymphocytic leukemia; CFU-c,
macrophage/granulocyte colony-forming units.

REFERENCES

1. Cavins, J.A., Kasakura, S., Thomas, E.D. and Ferrebee, J.W. Blood 20, 730 (1962).
2. Dicke, K.A., Spitzer, G., Peters, L., McCredie, K.B., Zander, A., Verma, D.S., Vellekoop, L. and Hester, J. The Lancet, March 10, 514 (1979).
3. Netzel, B., Rodt, H., Haas, R.J., Kolb, H.J. and Thierfelder, S. The Lancet, June 21, 1330 (1980).
4. Ritz, J., Bast, R.C., Jr., Clavell, L.A., Hercend, T., Sallan, S.E., Lipton, J.M., Feeney, M., Nathan, D.G. and Schlossman, S.F. Lancet, July 10, 60 (1982).
5. Murphy, S. B., Cancer Treat. Rep. 61, 1161 (1977).
6. Forster, H.K., Gudat, F.G., Girard, M.D., Albrecht, R., Schmidt, J., Ludwig, C. and Obrecht, J.P. Cancer Res. 42, 1927 (1982).

QUESTIONS AND ANSWERS

RITZ: Is 600 rads a marrow ablative dose in these patients?

BAUMGARTNER: I would not say that it is marrow ablative, but it is sufficient for these B cell lymphomas.

RITZ: I notice that you have a very rapid reconstitution in these patients and I wonder if this is coming from the marrow you added back or from the residual marrow?

BAUMGARTNER: Of course we would like to think that reconstitution is due to the marrow we add back, but it is very difficult to give a precise answer to this question.

The Future

Magic Bullets

THE USE OF IMMUNOTOXINS FOR THE TREATMENT OF CANCER[1]

Jonathan W. Uhr
Ellen S. Vitetta

Department of Microbiology
University of Texas Health Science Center
Dallas, Texas

I. INTRODUCTION

The term immunotoxin will be used to designate a hybrid molecule, one portion of which is a toxic protein and the other portion of which is an antibody or antigen. There are three major ways that immunotoxins can be used for the therapy of cancer: 1) in vitro treatment of bone marrow to delete cancer cells or T lymphocytes as part of the bone marrow transplantation approach; 2) parenteral treatment of patients bearing cancers; 3) parenteral treatment of cancer patients to modulate their immune response for therapeutic purposes.

Before discussing these approaches, we will present some background information about immunotoxins. The majority of current research in this field using toxic proteins is being performed with the plant toxin, ricin, and the problems associated with using ricin or its toxic subunit are in large measure similar to those using other protein toxins. We will focus, therefore, on studies utilizing ricin.

The working hypothesis by which ricin intoxicates a cell is shown in Figure 1. The concept is derived from earlier studies of others (1-5). The two points to be made are that endocytosis and translocation of the A chain across a membrane of an endocytic vesicle are considered essential steps. The precise mechanism by which the A chain of ricin gains access

---

[1]These studies were supported by NIH grants AI-11851 and CA-23115.

to the cytoplasm is not known. There is considerable evidence
from earlier studies of others (5) that the B chain plays a
role in the translocation. It is not surprising, therefore,
that conjugates of intact ricin and antibody are usually more
toxic than similar conjugates of antibody and highly purified
A chain. The other general points are that our own studies
involve immunoglobulin on B cells as the target antigen and
usually employ heterologous affinity-purified specific antibody. B cell surface Ig crosslinked by high affinity antibody
is known to be rapidly endocytosed and metabolized.

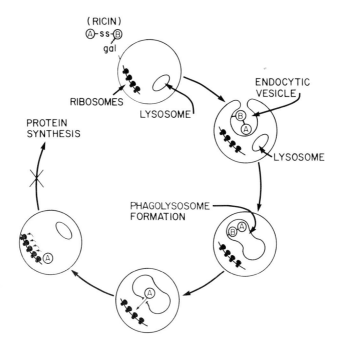

FIGURE 1. A model for the cytotoxic action of ricin (17).

II. RESULTS AND DISCUSSION

The first approach is the use of immunotoxins to kill tumor cells in infiltrated bone marrow as a step in the autologous bone marrow rescue approach in the treatment of cancer (reviewed in 6). Patients whose tumor cells show a steep dose-response curve in vitro to x-irradiation are potential candidates for this approach. The idea is to remove bone marrow during the first remission after chemotherapy and/or x-irradiation and to store the patient's marrow in the frozen state. If the patient relapses, the possibility of cure becomes minimal; hence, drastic therapy is indicated. The patient is then treated with supralethal doses of x-irradiation and/or chemotherapy and is rescued by the subsequent intravenous infusion of his/her own bone marrow. There are two major problems with this approach: the complete eradication of disease in vivo by the supralethal therapy and the need to eradicate occult tumor cells in the bone marrow. We reported approximately one year ago in a murine leukemia system (7) that, in the majority of cases, immunotoxins could kill virtually all leukemic cells in infiltrated murine bone marrow and suggested, therefore, that this approach would represent a major possibility for the clinical utilization of immunotoxins. These studies were performed using a B cell leukemia, BCL_1, described by Slavin and Strober (8) and anti-Ig-A chain immunotoxin. We emphasized that tumor-specific antibody was unnecessary and that the only specificity required is to use an antibody that reacts with the tumor cells and kills them, but does not react with the pluripotential stem cells which reconstitute the entire hematopoietic system.

We want to report two new findings along these lines which fortify our prediction concerning the usefulness of this approach. The first is a further follow-up of the earlier experiment reported in Nature (7) (Figure 2). We showed initially that at twelve weeks after transfer of the infiltrated and treated bone marrow, 17 of 20 animals were alive and appeared tumor-free. This is at the time when a single viable tumor cell injected into a virgin animal will produce overt clinical tumor in approximately 50% of the animals. Since that time we have followed such animals for an additional 13 weeks and we have done cell-transfer studies of blood and tissues from the treated animals to normal recipients. Of particular interest is the fact that an additional animal came down with leukemia at approximately 17 weeks after treatment, beyond the time that we would have

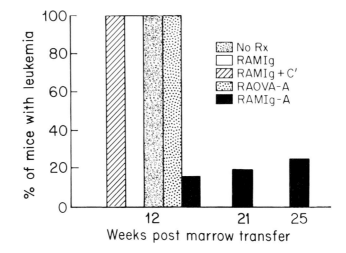

FIGURE 2.   Adoptive transfer into lethally irradiated
recipients of BCL_1-containing bone marrow cells treated with
rabbit anti-mouse Ig-A chain (RAMIg-A).   Bone marrow cells,
containing 10-15% tumor cells, were injected into groups of 20
mice at 10^6 marrow cells per mouse.   Every two weeks after
adoptive transfer, mice were examined for leukemia.   At 25
weeks, all surviving mice were sacrificed and 10^6 spleen cells
were adoptively transferred into normal recipients.   The
spleen cells from one of the mice caused tumor in these
recipients 10 weeks later.   Thus, this mouse is scored as
'leukemic' at 25 weeks (17).   RAOVA-A = rabbit anti-
ovalbumin-A chain.

detected disease from a single tumor cell growing in a virgin
animal.   In addition, at 25 weeks after treatment, cells were
transferred to normal recipients in order to detect occult
tumor cells that were present but undetected by flow cytometry
and presumably not growing.   All the transfers were negative
except for one animal which, although it appeared tumor-free,

could transfer leukemia from virtually all its tissues into normal animals. Therefore, the simplest interpretation of this experiment is that tumor cells were eradicated in approximately 75% of the animals. In three animals tumor appeared at precisely the time that one or two remaining cells would have evolved into clinical disease in non-immune animals. In two animals, tumor cells had not been eradicated, but their growth was suppressed by a host immune response. This response could be an active response in these animals to the injection of killed tumor cells in the bone marrow innoculum that had been treated with immunotoxin or it could have come from the transfer of a very small number of tumor-reactive T or pre-B cells present in such bone marrow.

Another new finding derives from studies with human bone marrow. The study was designed to determine the efficacy of immunotoxins in killing human neoplastic B cells selectively in the presence of human bone marrow. The studies were performed in collaboration with Dr. Michael Muirhead, Dr. Paul Martin and Dr. Beverly Torok-Storb (9). We mixed the Burkitt lymphoma B cell line, Daudi, with normal human marrow and attempted to kill the leukemic cells with polyvalent anti-human Ig-A chain immunotoxins without killing stem cells capable of reconstituting the hematopoietic system in humans. In these experiments, the A chains contained no detectable B chain as judged by the fact that 1mg of A chain was not lethal for mice. The lethal dose for an adult mouse is 300ng intact ricin. In contrast to the mouse, there is no assay in the human for the pluripotential stem cell, but there are in vitro cloning techniques for the slightly more mature stem cells for myeloid and erythroid lineages. The results of these experiments (shown in Table 1) indicate that 97-99% of colony-forming Daudi cells were killed, with no killing of myeloid/granulocyte colony-forming cells. Additional experiments indicated that these same immunotoxins had no effect on erythroid burst-forming unit (BFU_e) and erythroid colony-forming unit (CFU_e) stem cells of the erythrocytic lineage. We conclude that, using such immunotoxins, highly effective killing can be achieved with no detrimental effect on hematopoietic colony-forming cells. It is a reasonable assumption that there would be no detrimental effect on the pluripotential stem cell either. The extent of killing of neoplastic cells under the conditions employed (an incubation time of 20 minutes at 4°C) is encouraging. Since earlier stages of B cell lineages have been incriminated in the neoplastic process in spontaneous B cell malignancies in man, it would be advisable to use, in addition to anti-immunoglobulin immunotoxins, immunotoxins containing monoclonal antibodies against various B cell differentiation

antigens including those present on pre-B cells. We suggest,
therefore, that a cocktail of such antibody-A chain immunotoxins may offer the greatest likelihood of eradicating all
neoplastic B cells in human bone marrow, and we are optimistic
about the potential usefulness of immunotoxins in this
approach to the treatment of certain types of cancer.

How does this approach compare to others for eradicating
tumor cells in the bone marrow? We suggest tht the use of
immunotoxins may have advantages over the use of complement-
mediated cell killing for two reasons: 1) we do not believe
complement-mediated killing will be as effective as
immunotoxin-mediated killing after the latter approach is
further developed; 2) complement is frequently toxic for human
colony-forming cells, hence the problem of screening and
standardization will be very difficult compared to the
potential standardization of immunotoxins.

Another possible approach is to use immunotoxins composed
of intact ricin in the presence of high concentrations of
galactose in order to inhibit the nonspecific killing effect
of ricin while maintaining specific killing of the tumor
cells. This approach was used successfully in a rat leukemia
by Thorpe and his co-workers (10). Indeed, they emphasized
that these conjugates were far more effective in killing tumor
cells than A chain-containing immunotoxins. Hence, these
conjugates offer a major advantage in potency over A chain
conjugates. There are, however, problems with the use of
immunotoxins containing intact ricin: 1) ricin-containing
immunotoxins can damage stem cells; addition of galactose can
increase the 'window' of the therapeutic effect, but the
potential for such damage is present and is of concern; 2)
ricin transferred into the recipient of the bone marrow
transfer could be a problem if the inhibition by galactose of
nonspecific binding is not successful; 3) the general
deployment of ricin-containing conjugates to laboratories
carries with it certain responsibilities and risks which would
be attractive to avoid. Nevertheless, we believe this is a
viable alternative approach and clinical trials using immunotoxins containing either ricin or A chain will be important in
making decisions about which method is optimal in which
clinical situation.

There is a second approach to the bone marrow rescue
maneuver and that is the use of allogeneic bone marrow,
obviously tumor-free, in which mature T cells are removed by
treatment with anti-T cell immunotoxins. This has been accom-
plished in mice by Vallera et al. (11) using anti-Thy1 immunotoxins containing ricin. If this approach can be used
successfully in histoincompatible humans, it might supercede
the use of autologous marrow for treatment of cancer and also
be applicable for non-neoplastic diseases as well (in parti-

TABLE 1.   Soft Agar Cloning of Parallel Cultures of Daudi Cells and Bone Marrow Cells Following Treatment with Immunotoxin[+] (9)

Experiment	Cells	Treatment	Colonies*
1	Daudi	None	4550
		RαOVA-A	4970 ± 737
		RαHλκ-A	36 ± 24
	BM**	None	168 ± 40
		RαOVA-A	268 ± 63
		RαHλκ-A	248 ± 42
2	Daudi	None	138
		RαOVA-A	330
		RαHλκ-A	1 ± 1
	BM	None	359 ± 64
		RαOVA-A	359 ± 33
		RαHλκ-A	457 ± 21
3	Daudi	None	1010 ± 277
		RαOVA-A	698 ± 73
		RαHλκ-A	0 ± 0
	BM	None	370 ± 83
		RαOVA-A	399 ± 116
		RαHλκ-A	677 ± 53

[+] 2×10^4 Daudi cells or 5×10^5 bone marrow (BM) cells were plated out in soft agar in each dish. The numbers listed represent the mean colony counts per dish obtained from each treatment group. Most of the treatment groups contained three dishes, which were counted for colonies, and the mean colony count ± S.D. is given. Otherwise, the mean count from 2 dishes is given. In the first experiment RαOVA-A and RαHλK-A were used at a concentration of 12μg/ml. In experiments 2 and 3, the concentration of antibody-A chain was 25μg/ml.
*   Bone marrow assayed for granulocyte/macrophage-CFU exclusively.
**   Each experiment utilized a different bone marrow donor.
     RαOVA-A = rabbit anti-ovalbumin-A chain;
     RαHλK-A = rabbit anti-human λ,κ-A chain.

cular, aplastic anemia). One problem with this approach is that the recipient may not regain full immunocompetence. It is not yet proven that immunologic chimeras can respond normally to third-party antigens. On the other hand, there is evidence that such chimeras may have some anti-leukemic immunity as an added dividend (12-13).

A second use of immunotoxins is to administer them systemically to tumor-bearing individuals. In contrast to the use of immunotoxins for the in vitro treatment of bone marrow, systemic administration demands much stricter tumor cell specificity (i.e., cross-reactivity with normal cells may not be acceptable). In addition, information is needed about the pharmacokinetics of the immunotoxins and, in particular, their therapeutic index. Ideally, one would like to begin clinical trials with immunotoxins after the reagents have been optimized (that is, after determining conditions for preparing immunotoxins of the highest potency and the lowest toxicity). We have used anti-idiotype-A chain conjugates to treat mice bearing far-advanced BCL_1 tumors. In these mice, approximately 10^{10} tumor cells, or 20% of their body weight, was tumor. Our strategy was to nonspecifically reduce the tumor mass by at least 95% and try to kill the remainder of the cells with anti-idiotype-A chain conjugates. Nonspecific cytoreduction was carried out using total lymphoid irradiation, as developed by Kaplan and co-workers (14), and splenectomy. This regimen succeeded in producing a prolonged remission (that is, the mice appeared tumor-free twelve weeks later). The results were impressive, in that control animals treated with nontumor-reactive immunotoxins were all dead seven weeks after completion of the total lymphoid irradiation and splenectomy. It was of particular interest that we could reproduce these results with anti-delta (specific anti-IgD) immunotoxins. In a sense, this maneuver could be considered a step backward since we were using a normal cell surface molecule as our target antigen. On the other hand, it was very attractive for several reasons: 1) anti-delta is a more universal reagent than anti-idiotype since it is detectable on more than one-half of B cell tumors in man; 2) IgD is present on the surface of BCL_1 cells, although in very small amounts (probably less than an average of 5,000 molecules/cell); 3) there is very little IgD in the serum of man or mouse; 4) affinity-purified heterologous anti-delta is more easily prepared in large amounts than purified anti-idiotype antibody. Therefore, anti-human delta-A chain immunotoxins might be useful in systemic immunotherapy of human B cell tumors.

The results also show that three months after treatment with anti-delta immunotoxin, which should have eliminated normal IgD^+ lymphocytes, normal levels of IgD^+ cells are present. They had been reconstituted from stem cells, pre-B cells or IgM^+ IgD^- cells. In this particular instance, the price of killing BCL_1 cells, which was the killing of virtually all virgin B lymphocytes for a period of time, was acceptable. Serum antibodies and memory cells that lack surface IgD apparently provided the animal with sufficient immunity to survive during this interim period.

We have followed animals treated in this fashion for a longer period of time than previously published to determine if remission persisted and, if so, whether the animals were tumor-free or whether there was an immune response keeping a small number of tumor cells in check. The answers to these questions are that the remissions appear to be very prolonged, since we have followed animals for twenty-five weeks and they remained well and tumor-free clinically. However, when cells from the tissues of such animals were transferred to normal recipients, they invariably caused tumor in the recipients. We conclude, therefore, that the mice in prolonged remission were not tumor-free. We suspect that a host immune response to the small number of remaining tumor cells was sufficient to cope with the tumor. This putative host immune response may be an anti-idiotypic one.

This last observation emphasizes again the critical nature of the host immune response in the tumor-host relationship and raises the final possibility that one major potential of these reagents is the modulation of the immune response for thera- peutic purposes. One immediate problem facing the use of monoclonal antibodies in human therapy is the potential immune response of the human against the mouse monoclonal antibody. Even the use of human antibodies may not alleviate this problem because of the possibility that humans will make an anti-idiotypic response against human monoclonal antibody. Indeed, the response in patients against mouse monoclonal antibodies used thus far frequently has an anti-idiotypic component (15). We, therefore, have attempted to induce immunologic tolerance in an adoptive transfer system as a prelude to using immunotoxins composed of antigen-A chain conjugates to induce immunologic tolerance in vivo to foreign proteins. Thus, we have taken splenic cells from mice immunized many weeks previously with dinitrophenol-keyhole limpet hemocyanin (DNP-KLH) in complete Freund's adjuvant. We incubated their splenic cells with antigen-containing immuno- toxins, namely trinitrophenol-human serum albumin (TNP-HSA)-A chain and a control immunotoxin (human serum albumin-A chain) (HSA-A chain) or nothing, and then transferred the washed cells into irradiated recipients that were challenged with TNP-sheep red blood cells (SRBC). The A chain preparations contained 0.2–0.8% B chains as judged by their LD_{50} in mice and by radioimmunoassay. The serum antibody titers 1-4 weeks later showed that the response to TNP (DNP and TNP cross-react extensively at the antibody level) in those recipients that received cells exposed to DNP-containing immunotoxins was reduced more than 95%, whereas the response to SRBC in such recipients was normal (Figure 3). In addition, neither the control immunotoxin (HSA-A chain) nor antigen itself (TNP-HSA) had any effect on either the anti-TNP or the anti-SRBC response. Additional experiments showed that similar results were obtained when purified B cells rather than spleen cells were used. Thus, it appears that specific immune unresponsiveness can be induced in B cells in vitro with immunotoxins. Obviously, we are interested in whether such results can be obtained in vivo and in the duration of the subsequent unresponsiveness. Should the unresponsiveness wane, we would likewise be interested in the effect of repeated injections of immunotoxins on the reduction of unresponsiveness.

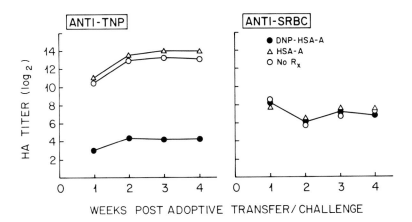

FIGURE 3. Serum hemagglutination titer (HA) of irradiated mice injected with 10^7 cells treated as indicated. Spleen cells were obtained from mice previously injected with DNP-KLH and SRBC. Cells were treated for 15 hrs at 4°C with immunotoxin ($50\mu g/10^6$ cells), control immunotoxin or nothing (see text). 10^7 cells were injected into irradiated mice. These mice were injected with antigen two hours later and the hemagglutination titer of the sera evaluated 1-4 weeks later. Although not shown in the figure, inoculation of cells with antigen alone had no effect on their subsequent responsiveness in vivo (17).

Similar in vitro studies have been performed by Volkman et al. (16) using intact ricin conjugated to tetanus toxoid in a human in vitro system containing galactose to prevent non-specific killing. This approach would not be applicable in vivo because of the toxicity of ricin.

The usefulness of inducing tolerance in vivo obviously extends beyond that of treating cancer patients with mono-clonal antibodies, and could also be useful for treatment of autoimmune disease, preventing transplantation rejection, etc. With regard to cancer, it might be possible to modulate the immune response to cancer in a favorable way by using immuno-toxins specific to particular subsets of lymphocytes. More information is needed about the subsets of lymphocytes that are responsible for immunity to particular tumors as well as the cellular subsets and cytokines involved in the activation and regulation of such subsets. Once such insight is avail-able, it might be possible to increase tumor immunity by appropriate administration of immunotoxins to delete a suppressor subset or a subset that secretes a blocking anti-body.

To summarize, the use of immunotoxins in the bone marrow rescue approach is probably the most likely to yield positive results at this point in time. In the long run, parenterally administered immunotoxins may be useful not only in killing tumor cells but also in preventing antibody responses to mono-clonal antibodies and in increasing tumor immunity.

ACKNOWLEDGMENTS

We thank Mr. Y. Chen, Ms. L. Trahan, Ms. C. Bockhold and Mr. T. Tucker for expert technical assistance and Ms. F. Hall for secretarial help.

ABBREVIATIONS

BFU_e, erythroid burst-forming units; CFU_e, erythroid colony-forming units; DNP, dinitrophenol; KLH, keyhole limpet hemocyanin; TNP, trinitrophenol; HSA, human serum albumin; SRBC, sheep red blood cells.

REFERENCES

1. Olsnes, S. and Pihl, A., in 'Pharmacology of Bacterial
    Toxins' (J. Drews and F. Dornes, eds.), Pergamon Press,
    New York, in press.
2. Olsnes, S. and Pihl, A. Biochemistry 12, 3121 (1973).
3. Olsnes, S., Sandvig, K., Refsnes, K., and Pihl, A.
    J. Biol Chem. 257, 3985 (1976).
4. Thorpe, P.E. and Ross, W.C.J.   Immunol. Rev. 62, 119
    (1982).
5. Neville, D.M., Jr. and Youle, R.J.   Immunol. Rev. 62, 75
    (1982).
6. Gale, R.P. J. Amer. Med. Assoc. 243, 540 (1980).
7. Krolick, K.A., Uhr, J.W., Vitetta, E.S. Nature 295, 604
    (1982).
8. Slavin, S. and Strober, S. Nature 272, 624 (1977).
9. Muirhead, M., Martin, P.J., Torok-Storb, B., Uhr, J.W.
    and Vitetta, E.S. Blood, in press.
10. Thorpe, P.E., Mason, D.W., Brown, A.N.F., Simmonds, S.J.,
    Ross, W.C.J., Cumber, A.J. and Forrester, J.A. Nature
    297, 594 (1982).
11. Vallera, D.A., Youle, R.J., Neville, D.M., Jr.,
    Kersey, J.H. J. Exp. Med. 155, 949 (1982).
12. Bortin, M.M., Truitt, R.L. and Rimm, A.A. Nature 281,
    1979 (1979).
13. Weiden, P.L., Flournoy, N., Thomas, E.D., Prentic, R.,
    Fefer, A., Buckner, C.D. and Storb, R. New Eng. J. Med.
    300, 1068 (1979).
14. Kaplan, H.S., in 'Hodgkin's Disease,' 2nd ed.
    (M. Chastain, ed.), Harvard Univ. Press, Cambridge, MA,
    (1980).
15. Levy, R., Miller, R.N., Stratte, P., Maloney, D.G.,
    Link, M., Meeker, T.C., Oseroff, A., Thielemans, K. and
    Warnke, R., in 'Monoclonal Antibodies and Cancer'
    (Proceedings of the IV Armand Hammer Cancer Symposium)
    (B.D. Boss, R.E. Langman, I.S. Trowbridge and R.
    Dulbecco, eds.), Academic Press, New York, in press.
16. Volkman, D.J., Ahmed, A., Fauce, A.S. and Neville, D.M.,
    Jr. J. Exp. Med. 156, 634 (1982).
17. Vitetta, E.S., Krolick, K.A., Miyama-Inaba, M.,
    Cushley, W. and Uhr, J.W. Science 219, 644 (1983).

QUESTIONS AND ANSWERS

CHEN: Is the microenvironment at the site of immunotoxin binding conducive to T cell activation and hence the generation of normal immune elimination of tumor cells?

UHR: While we have no specific information relevant to your question, it is a possibility.

RITZ: Have you made a specific comparison between monoclonal and polyvalent anti-immunoglobulins conjugated with ricin A chain?

UHR: Essentially all the work I have described here was carried out with a polyvalent rabbit anti-immunoglobulin that had been affinity purified. Perhaps Dr. Vitetta could add to this.

VITTETA: We did compare a monoclonal anti-delta, H.10.4.22, which has a rather high affinity, to the polyvalent rabbit serum in our in vitro system and found little to distinguish them. However, we have not made an in vivo comparison.

NEVILLE: I wonder if you know how much B chain contamination there is in your ricin A chain preparations, because you have better results than we can get with our A chain preparations.

UHR: It varies. For example, in the experiment with Daudi, where cells were killed to virtually 100%, we could not detect any biological B chain activity even when 1mg was injected into a mouse. Of course, in no case could we detect B chain biochemically, but this is a crude assay which would not detect a 1% contamination. I don't think there is any question that, as A chain is purified, cytotoxicity decreases and addition of B chain can restore this loss. However, it is clear that significant toxicity can be achieved with A chain alone, as shown by the Daudi results. We, like everybody else, worry about the unpredictability of the potency of a given A chain-immunoglobulin conjugate. Hopefully, the paper by Dr. Thorpe will go a long way towards helping here.

TROWBRIDGE: In general, the in vivo therapeutic effects of ricin A-antibody conjugates given immediately to animals challenged with graded doses of tumor cells have been much less effective than you have observed with the clinical BCL_1 model of cytoreductive therapy. Have you directly tested the effects of ricin A-anti-Ig antibody immediately after inoculation of graded doses of cells?

UHR: No.

OLDHAM: Along similar lines, do you know the maximum number of tumor cells that can be erradicated under optimal conditions?

UHR: No.

LANDY: There has been a long-standing controversy regarding the putative role of cytotoxic T cells in the rejection of allogeneic bone marrow. Since Uhr et al. now have the capability (via idiotypic-immunotoxins) to selectively eliminate this category of cell from marrow, I ask whether such altered allogeneic marrow becomes readily engrafted; i.e., can selectively depleted marrow restore immune competence?

UHR: We have not performed that experiment, but it has been done by Madeline Kersey and looked a very successful experiment.

IMMUNOTOXINS

Hildur E. Blythman, Pierre Casellas,
Olivier Gros, Franz K. Jansen,
Jean-Claude Laurent, Gilbert Richer,
and Hubert Vidal

Centre de Recherches Clin-Midy
34082 Montpellier
FRANCE

I. INTRODUCTION

The idea of using a carrier to convey drugs to target tissues is not new, as Ehrlich at the turn of the century had proposed a sort of 'magic bullet' to attain specific targets. However, the idea materialized only around 1958, when Mathé and his collaborators prepared the first conjugate, using specific antibodies to which methotrexate was chemically linked (1).

Mathé had many followers. In 1970, Moolten and Cooperband described a variation on the theme, preparing a conjugate using diphtheria toxin instead of a drug (2). But whole toxins have one drawback. Most are made of two chains or domains: the B chain which binds to sugars on most cells, and the A (or active) chain which enters the cytoplasm to exert its toxic effect at the level of the protein-synthesizing system (3). Consequently, other groups developed the idea using only the toxic moiety of the whole toxin in order to increase the specificity of the conjugate by eliminating the nonspecific binding B domain, which would otherwise stick to all cells regardless of their antigenic characteristics.

II. RESULTS AND DISCUSSION

In our laboratory, a great effort was dedicated to
increase the efficiency of these conjugates (which we call
immunotoxins) (4) by attempting to obtain a very highly purified A chain of the plant toxin ricin. Combining ion-exchange
with affinity chromatography, using DEAE-Sepharose, we managed
to produce an extremely pure A chain which shows an in vitro
activity between 2000 and one million times lower than native
ricin, depending on the cell line tested (5). An accessory
finding, when several cell lines were compared, is the fact
that the toxicity of ricin does not correlate with that of its
purified A chain (5). The degree of purity of our A chain is
shown by the fact that we were able to obtain crystals (Figure
1).

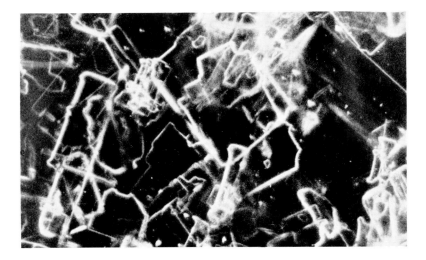

FIGURE 1. Ricin A chain crystals.

Upon approaching the construction of immunotoxins, we
considered that when replacing the B chain by any given antibody, the bond holding together both moieties of this hybrid
molecule should imitate the natural linkage. Therefore, by
several steps the A chain was bound to the antibody, creating
an S-S bridge, which is the type of linkage found in native
ricin.

Several antibodies were used, allowing us to employ different antigenic models. First we used hapten-labeled cells (TNP-HeLa, TNP-L1210, TNP-WEHI-7) to test an anti-trinitrophenol (TNP) immunotoxin (4). A second model was the Thy1.2 mouse differentiation antigen tested with the mouse leukemia WEHI-7 (6). Then, a human T cell differentiation antigen (T65) was chosen, using as test cells MOLT-4, CEM (5), RPMI-8402 or Ichikawa cells. Finally, a human melanoma system was used, the P97 antigen described by Hellström et al. (7) and found on SK-Mel 28 cells (8) (Figure 2). Immunotoxin activity was tested in vitro, incubating target and control cells for varying lengths of time in the presence of either immunotoxin (IT), native ricin, its purified A chain or non-specific IT (last two as negative controls).

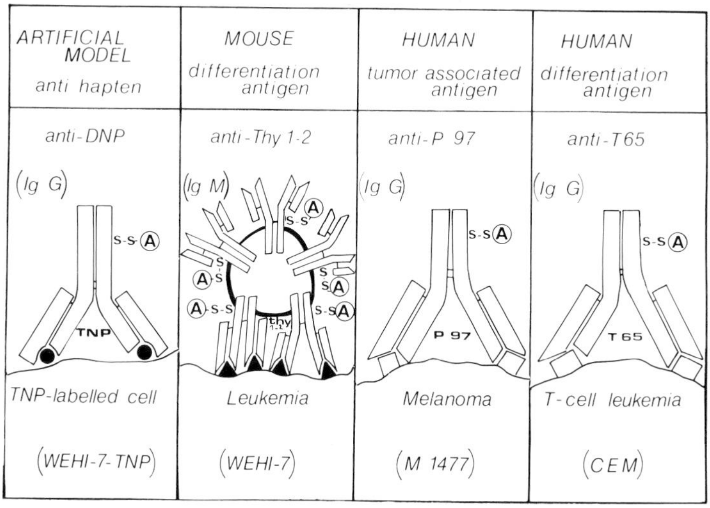

FIGURE 2. Different antigenic specificities used for immunotoxin models.

One finding which became evident when different models were compared was that the specificity factor (ratio of the concentration needed for 50% cytotoxicity with A chain or

unrelated IT and the concentration required for 50% cytotoxity
with specific IT or ricin) when using natural antigen models
was lower than that of intact ricin. The other apparent difference was a different slope of the curve, so that extremely
high IT concentrations were needed to reach near 100% cytotoxicity (Figure 3).

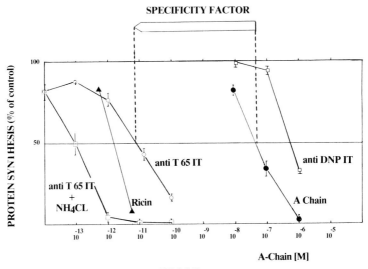

FIGURE 3. Effect of NH_4Cl on anti-T65 immunotoxin tested
on human T-leukemia cells. IT = immunotoxin; DNP =
dinitrophenol.

Considering the implications of an in vivo application of
this molecule, another method was chosen to verify the
efficacy of the cytotoxic effects of IT. Once cells had been
exposed to IT for a certain incubation time, they were plated
and further incubated to allow for any cell surviving the IT
treatment to grow and give rise to a colony (5). A specific
killing index was defined as being the ratio between the
concentration of A chain killing 0% of cells and the concentration of IT killing 100% of target cells. In the case of
anti-P97 IT (on SK-Mel 28 cells), the specific killing index
found was consistently 30. Thus, it became evident that the
IT molecule needed an activation or potentiation effect. As a

result, several products were investigated, and it was found that NH_4Cl exerted a potentiating effect which could be shown by both in vitro methods. Using NH_4Cl as activator, the specific killing index for anti-P97 IT was 300 (5). This specific killing index also expresses the security margin, which shows that free A chain, if liberated in vivo, has to greatly accumulate before nontarget cells would be damaged.

Another aspect of the IT approach to cancer therapy which we have been studying recently is the kinetics of IT activity. It became apparent that this was an important factor when cells were incubated with a single IT dose for different lengths of time. Although 50% cell killing could be reached quite early (12 hrs for anti-Thy 1.2 IT, for example), the time needed for 100% killing was reached very late if at all (with anti-T 65 IT, after more than 40 hrs of incubation, the maximum cytotoxicity obtained was 80%). In the presence of 10mM NH_4Cl, the kinetics of killing of both IT anti-P97 and anti-T65 were greatly accelerated and were comparable to that of ricin (8).

The implications of this phenomenon are easy to envisage. The main advantage is to be able to induce a fast killing of target cells, which is one way of overcoming cellular multiplication. As a consequence, a successful elimination of residual tumor cells could most probably be obtained in a clinical situation.

Another aspect of the study of ITs was to compare the disulfide bridge to a thioether bond; under some conditions the former is labile whereas the latter is not. We found that, while a disulfide bridge produces an active molecule, a stable thioether bridge shows no activity in vitro (Figure 4). This is not surprising, as the native ricin contains a disulfide bond. Recent results on the pharmacokinetics of IT show that the half-life of a disulfide-linked IT is on the order of 4.5 hours, whereas conjugates with a thioether bridge persist much longer in circulation (more than 8 hours).

Despite all the limiting factors of ITs which are presently under study in our laboratory, we have been able to demonstrate that they have in vivo activity. Using the anti-T65 IT, we obtained an increased survival of nude mice receiving i.p. $25x10^6$ Ichikawa cells (a human T cell leukemia, kindly provided by Dr. Shaw Watanabe) (9) followed by an 8-day i.p. treatment with specific IT as compared to free A chain plus antibody (T101) (10). Figure 5 shows the results of this preliminary experiment: a delay of fourteen days could be determined at the 50% survival times and an overall difference of twenty days at 100% death. These results, although far from satisfactory, are encouraging, and we hope that by

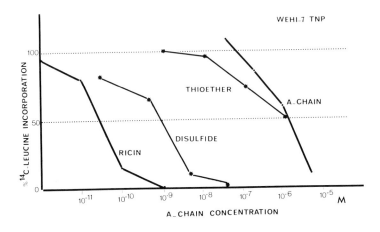

FIGURE 4. Comparison of the activity of two anti-DNP immunotoxins on TNP-labeled WEHI-7 murine leukemia cells.

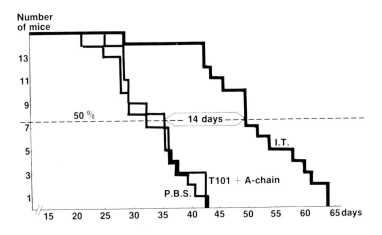

FIGURE 5. Effect of an anti-T65 (T101) immunotoxin on the survival of nude mice after injection of human T leukemia (Ichikawa) cells.

improving the activity by any of the means mentioned earlier a much better result can be expected.

Another approach to immunotherapy with IT is being proposed by several laboratories. We also expect to obtain significant results with the in vitro application of IT to treat tumor-contaminated bone marrow, both in the autologous as well as the allogeneic situations (expecting to eliminate either residual leukemic cells in the first case or T cells capable of generating an undesirable graft-versus-host disease in the second case). This approach is currently being investigated in our laboratory.

ABBREVIATIONS

TRP, trinitrophenol; IT, immunotoxin.

REFERENCES

1. Mathé, G., Loc, T.B., and Bernard, J.   Cr. Acad. Sci. (Paris) 246, 1626 (1958).
2. Moolten, F.L. and Cooperband, S.   Science 169, 68 (1970).
3. Olsnes, S. and Pihl, A.   Biochemistry 12, 3121 (1973).
4. Jansen, F.K., Blythman, H.E., Carrière, D., Diaz, J., Gros, P., Hennequin, J.R., Paolucci, F., Pau, B., Poncelet, P., Richer, G., Salhi, S.L., Vidal, H., and Voisin, G.A. Immunol. Letters 2, 97 (1980).
5. Jansen, F.K., Blythman, H.E., Carrière, D., Gros, O., Gros, P., Laurent, J.C., Paolucci, F., Pau, B., Poncelet, P., Richer, G., Vidal, H., Voisin, G.A.   Immunol. Rev. 62, 185 (1982).
6. Blythman, H.E., Casellas, P., Gros, O., Gros, P., Jansen, F.K., Paolucci, F., Pau, B., and Vidal, H.   Nature 290, 145 (1981).
7. Hellström, I., Brown, J.P., and Hellström, K.E. J. Immunol. 127, 157 (1981).
8. Casellas, P., Brown, J.P., Gros, O., Gros, P., Hellström, I., Jansen, F.K., Poncelet, P., Roncucci, R., Vidal, H., and Hellström, K.E.   Int. J. Cancer 30, 437 (1982).
9. Watanabe, S., Shimosato, Y., Kameya, T., Kuroki, M., Kitahara, T. Minato, K., and Shimoyama, M.   Cancer Res. 38, 3494 (1978).
10. Royston, I., Majda, J.A., Yamamoto, G.Y. et al., in 'Protides of the Biological Fluids, 28th Colloquium' (H. Peeters, ed.), p. 537. Pergamon Press, New York (1980).

QUESTIONS AND ANSWERS

VITETTA: Does NH_4Cl enhance killing by control immunotoxin?

BLYTHMAN: No,   the NH_4Cl affects   only   the   specific
immunotoxin.

VITETTA: Does NH_4Cl change the rate of internalization of
immunotoxin from the cell surface?

BLYTHMAN: We have not looked into the details yet, because
there are many possibilities which need to be carefully
evaluated.

MONOCLONAL ANTIBODY-RICIN CONJUGATES FOR THE TREATMENT OF GRAFT-VERSUS-HOST DISEASE: PRESENT AND FUTURE PROSPECTS

David M. Neville, Jr., Richard J. Youle,

Section on Biophysical Chemistry
Laboratory of Neurochemistry
National Institute of Mental Health
Bethesda, Maryland

John H. Kersey, and Daniel A. Vallera

Department of Therapeutic Radiology
and Laboratory of Medicine/Pathology
University of Minnesota
Minneapolis, Minnesota

I. INTRODUCTION

Six years ago our laboratory suggested that a new class of cell-type-specific toxic reagents could be constructed by altering the receptor specificity of toxins (1). Although the concept of drug targeting had been proposed much earlier by Ehrlich (2), our proposal was conceptually different in that it focused on the physiology of receptor-mediated protein transport systems which the toxins themselves exemplified (3). While this may seem like a minor distinction, it allowed us to define the problem mechanistically and thereby provided a theoretical framework for our research effort (4-7).

Today we are ready to begin clinical trials with three of the reagents which have been designed to eliminate T cell activity from human donor bone marrow allografts. It is our belief, based on animal studies (8-10), that these reagents will provide a reproducible clinical regimen, free from the difficulties of complement use, for the prevention of graft-versus-host disease (GVHD) following therapeutic allogeneic bone marrow transplantation (11). It is our hope that the use of these reagents will eventually permit human marrow transplantation across major histocompatibility barriers, a feat already possible in experimental animals (10,12-15). Alleviating the requirement for an HLA-matched sibling donor would greatly increase the number of patients with leukemia and aplastic anemia who could benefit from this therapy.

The exquisite selectivity of the targeting portion of our reagents has been made possible by the discovery of monoclonal antibody technology (16) and its application toward defining cell surface membrane differentiation antigens (17-19). The choice of using intact ricin in the presence of lactose for the toxin portion has been dictated by our knowledge about the role of the toxin B chain in facilitating efficient entry of the toxic A chain. This knowledge stems from basic research in toxin transport (20-24) and the use of toxin conjugates as mechanistic probes (7).

II. RESULTS

Three monoclonal IgG anti-human T cell antibody-ricin conjugates have been synthesized as previously described utilizing a thioether linkage (25). The monoclonal antibodies used and the molecular weights of their antigens are: TA-1, 170,000 plus 95,000 complex (26); T101, 65,000 (18); and UCHT1, 19,000 (27).

In order to compare the effects of these conjugates on T cells and bone marrow stem cells, we have incubated these conjugates for 2 hours at 37°C under identical conditions with Ficoll-Hypaque-purified peripheral blood mononuclear cells and bone marrow cells obtained by iliac crest taps. Stem cell activity was assayed by counting pluripotential or mixed colonies in semi-solid medium, using the mixed granulocyte, erythroid, macrophage, monocyte (CFU-GEMM) assay (28,29). In this assay all mixed colonies contain at least granulocytic and erythroid elements, a majority of colonies contain monocytes or macrophages and one-fifth of the colonies contain megakaryocytes (29). T cell activity was assayed by tritiated thymidine incorporation after phytohemagglutinin (PHA) stimulation.

The effects of the three conjugates on T cells and stem cells are shown in a recent paper by Vallera, et al. (30). All three conjugates, TA-1-ricin, T101-ricin, and UCHT1-ricin, inhibited the PHA response more than 90% at 300ng/ml. Assuming a molecular weight of the antibody-ricin conjugates as 210,000 for a 1:1 conjugate (consistent with high pressure liquid chromatography and gel electrophoresis data), the 300ng/ml dose would be 1.4×10^{-9}M. At the concentration of conjugate which inhibits T cells more than 90% (1.4×10^{-9}M) there is no significant inhibition of stem cells. A comparison of the dose of the conjugate which inhibits the T cells or stem cell response 50% shows that T101-ricin and UCHT1-ricin are 30-fold and TA-1-ricin is 100-fold more toxic to T cells than stem cells. Erythroid burst-forming colonies (BFU-E) were equal or less sensitive to conjugate toxicity compared to CFU-GEMM colonies. The standard deviations are those between experiments and are generally equal to the deviations between triplicates within one experiment. The deviations are large in the CFU-GEMM assay owing to the small number of colonies counted per dish (12 ± 4).

The majority of human T cells carry the three determinants for TA-1, T101 and UCHT1. However, it is of some concern that subpopulations may exist which lack one or two of these determinants. T cell killing with a single conjugate could then reach a limiting value. In such cases, mixtures of conjugates could have additive effects (31). Another situation in which mixtures of conjugates would provide greater killing exists when receptor saturation of a single conjugate occurs (31). Calculations indicate that human peripheral T cell receptors for UCHT1-ricin are 50% saturated at 105ng/ml and 91% saturated at 1050ng/ml ($Kd = 5 \times 10^{-10}$M [27]). A similar calculation for TA-1-ricin gives 50% saturation at 210ng/ml ($Kd = 1 \times 10^{-9}$M, unpublished data).

When the effects of single conjugates and an equal part mixture of all three are compared by the inhibition of PHA response, plotted on a log scale, the results deviate from a single hit killing curve for each of the individual conjugates at 300ng/ml. This indicates that there is a resistant population seen at 300ng/ml. We cannot determine whether this resistance is due to a subset lacking one determinant, receptor saturation, or both phenomena. The mixture overcomes the resistance at 300ng/ml, providing a log linear dose response in the range of 30-300ng/ml. Therefore, we believe that conjugate mixtures offer the best theoretical and practical approach to reduce GVHD (30).

We are uncertain as to how many allogeneic T cells a human can tolerate. In mice, the incidence of GVHD is considerably reduced when infused allogenic T cells are in the range of 4×10^5/kg (8,32). If we wish to achieve this in humans when a typical human transplant consists of 2×10^8 nucleated cells/kg, 22% of which are T cells (33), then a T cell reduction in donor marrow of 10^{-2} is required. Using conjugate mixtures at 300ng/ml and the PHA assay, we seem to be in this range. However, the conversion of the PHA assay into units of fraction of surviving cells may be unreliable, because cell multiplication and death are nearly balanced under the conditions the assays are generally performed (34). Also, preliminary data using the mixed lymphocyte reaction (MLR) assay indicates that conjugate mixtures are more effective than individual conjugates, even though the reduction in T cell activity is not as great. The linearity of the MLR assay when used to judge T cell killing is also in question, because this assay is nonlinear when the ratio of responder to stimulator cells is varied (35).

It should also be pointed out that the in vitro stem cell assay may not accurately reflect the human in vivo toxicity dose response. Many factors govern toxin toxicity, such as intracellular toxin degradation and intracellular vesicle traffic (36), all of which may be influenced by the cellular environment. However, these in vitro studies provide quantitative starting points for clinical trials.

III. DISCUSSION

We will now briefly review the variables which affect conjugate killing of target and nontarget cells. We will present a model which can explain much of the perplexing data obtained with different types of conjugates. We believe this model is important because it points out a way that our present-day conjugates can be improved and also focuses on the areas where further basic investigations are required.

Some of the perplexing features of toxins such as ricin and diphtheria toxin (DT) are (1) a pronounced lag period which is dose dependent over a certain range, (2) variation in toxicity between cell types that is not always correlated with receptor number or affinity (39-41), and (3) deviations from single-hit killing curves before cell surface receptors are appreciably saturated (42,43).

Toxin conjugates with either monoclonal antibodies or other receptor binding moieties display the following interesting features: (1) conjugates with A chains are selective (44-48) but exhibit reduced killing capacity as compared to the parent toxin (8,49); (2) diphtheria toxin A chain is generally much poorer than ricin A chain in this respect (46,22,43); (3) toxin B chains enhance the killing of conjugates and in some cases this is a receptor-mediated process within the cell (6-8); and (4) some conjugates (perhaps all) do not exhibit lag periods (8).

It is our belief that features 1 and 3 are the major limitations to the in vivo use of antitumor monoclonal antibody-toxin conjugates today. In any therapeutic situation the ratio of nontarget to target cells will be in the range of 10^3-10^5, and nontarget cells will carry the toxin receptor located on the toxin B chain. If the B chain is included in the conjugate for efficient entry, then its extracellular binding activity must be blocked. Toxins such as ricin and diphtheria toxin inhibit protein synthesis when their enzymatically active A chains inactivate substrates only present in the cytosol compartment (50,51). Understanding how conjugates and toxins behave towards different cells can be reduced to understanding the flow of A chain from the external medium to the cytosol and then identifying the rate limiting step(s).

In Figure 1 the major compartments include the external medium (M), receptors (R) for toxins (R1), and alternate receptors for conjugate binding moieties such as T cell glycoprotein determinants (R3). Compartment B represents the lipid bilayer and C the cytosol. The flux from B to C depends on the concentration in B times a constant k''' ($F_{BC} = [B]K'''$). Receptors function to raise the concentration in B even when the concentration in M is low.

The major variables include, then, the flux from the medium to the receptor compartment (FMR_1), which is dependent on receptor affinity (K_A) and receptor number (N). Another major variable is k''', the rate constant governing flux from the bilayer to the cytosol, which is probably increased by hydrophobic residues, as suggested by Boquet et al., (21) and Uchida et al., (22). This accounts for the ricin A chain conjugates having greater toxicity than diphtheria A chain hybrids. In addition, B chains provide increased hydrophobicity. In this regard, DT CRM45, a B chain mutant which has retained hydrophobicity (21), behaves like ricin A chain (RTA).

However, B chains provide a higher flux than is accountable by simple hydrophobicity. This high degree of flux involves use of a second internal receptor which is unique to the toxin (6,7,42). To get from R1 to R2 some kind of processing is involved which, in the case of DT, is pH dependent (23,24). The time taken to process defines the lag period. In the mouse, which is highly resistant to DT, R1 is present (39-41) but cannot transfer toxin to R2. R2 can be reached from M, but only at higher concentrations (40). Flow from M→R2 also occurs in DT-sensitive animals and when ricin is present at high concentrations; this can be seen as a decrease in lag unaccompanied by an increase in the entry rate (43).

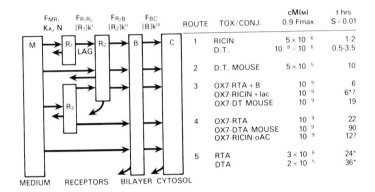

FIGURE 1. The flow of toxin A chains from the external medium to the cell cytosol compartment is modeled. Different toxins, toxin fragments or conjugates take different routes, which have varied entry efficiencies (see references). * indicates lack of saturation. ? indicates an extrapolation from other data. D.T. = diphtheria toxin; mouse = in the mouse system (relatively resistant to diphtheria toxin); OX7 = an anti-Thy1.1 monoclonal antibody; RTA = ricin toxin A chain; B = ricin B chain; lac = lactose; DTA = diphtheria toxin A chain; RICIN-oAC = o-acetylated ricin at the lactose binding site (6).

When conjugates contain B chains they enter at R3 and can interact with R2, achieving a higher flux than is possible via R3 → B. A chain conjugates, whose entry is enhanced by adding B chains separately, enter at R3, while B enters via R2 (no lag). B cannot enter at R1, because processing only occurs with intact toxin.

The routes used by a variety of toxins, toxin fragments and conjugates are listed in Figure 1. The entry rate (t) or log decrease protein synthesis/time is defined by the time taken to reach 1% of control protein synthesis under conditions in which the external receptor is 91% saturated (i.e., 10xKd). The concentration in the medium at which this occurs is called cM at $0.91F_{max}$ or the concentration at which the flux is 91% of the maximum value. A look at t, cM and N provides an overall view of the efficiency of the process for each substance.

Our analysis indicates that, by far, the most efficient entry route involves $R_1 \rightarrow R_2 \rightarrow B \rightarrow C$. Future work calls for constructing conjugates which enter at R_3 but proceed to R_1. Probably, the processing responsible for the lag has something to do with the high efficiency of this process. Approaches should be devised to have conjugates which can dissociate once internalized, freeing the toxin binding site to interact with R_1 and thus permitting the processing event. High efficiency conjugates with reversibly blocked toxin binding sites offer a rational methodology for achieving in vivo therapy of malignant tumors with toxin-monoclonal antibody conjugates.

ABBREVIATIONS

GVHD, graft-versus-host disease; CFU-GEMM, mixed (granulocyte, erythroid, macrophage, monocyte) colony-forming units; PHA, phytohemagglutinin; MLR, mixed lymphocyte reaction; DT, diphtheria toxin.

REFERENCES

1. Chang, T. and Neville, D.M., Jr. J. Biol. Chem. 252, 1505 (1977).
2. Himmelweit, F., in 'The Collected Papers of Paul Erlich' (F. Himmelweit, ed.), Vol. 3. Pergamon Press, New York (1960).
3. Neville, D.M., Jr., and Chang, T.M., in 'Current Topics in Membranes and Transport', (B. Bronner and A. Kleinzeller, eds.), Vol. 10, 65. Academic Press, New York (1978).
4. Youle, R.J. and Neville, D.M., Jr. J. Biol. Chem. 254, 11089 (1979).
5. Youle, R.J., Murray, G.J., and Neville, D.M., Jr. Proc. Natl. Acad. Sci. USA 76, 5559 (1979).
6. Youle, R.J., Murray, G.J., and Neville, D.M., Jr. Cell 23, 551 (1981).
7. Youle, R.J. and Neville, D.M., Jr. J. Biol. Chem. 257, 1598 (1982).
8. Korngold, R. and Sprent, J. J. Exp. Med 148, 1687 (1978).
9. Vallera, D.A., Soderling, C., and Kersey, J. Transplantation (Baltimore) 31, 218 (1981).

10. Vallera, D.A., Youle, R.J., Neville, D.M., Jr., and Kersey, J. J. Exp. Med. 155, 949 (1982).

11. Good, R., in 'Immunobiology' (R. A. Good, ed.), p. 231. S. M. Allen Associated, Connecticut (1971).

12. Muller-Ruchholtz, W., Wottage, H.V., and Muller-Hermelink, H.K. Transplant. Proc. 8, 537 (1976).

13. Truitt, R.L. and Pollard, M. Transplantation (Baltimore) 21, 12 (1976).

14. Muto, M., Sado, T., Aizawa, S., Kamisaku, H., and Kubo, E. J. Immunol. 127, 2421 (1981).

15. Vallera, D.A., Solderling, C., and Kersey, J.H. J. Immunol. 128, 218 (1982).

16. Williams, A.F., Galfre, G., and Milstein, C. Cell 12, 663 (1977).

17. Le Bien, T.W. and Kersey, J.H. J. Immunol. 125, 2208 (1980).

18. Royston, I., Majda, J.A., Baird, S.M. Meserve, B.L., and Griffiths, J.C. J. Immunol. 125, 725 (1980).

19. Beverly, P.C.L. and Callard, R.E. Eur. J. Immunol. 11, 329 (1981).

20. Boquet, P., Silverman, M.S., Pappenheimer, A.M., Jr., and Vernon, W.B. Proc. Natl. Acad. Sci. USA 73, 4449 (1976).

21. Uchida, T., Mekada, E., and Okada, Y. J. Biol. Chem. 255, 6687 (1980).

22. Draper, R.K. and Simon, M.I. Cell 87, 849 (1980).

23. Sandvig, K. and Olsnes, S. J. Biol. Chem. 256, 9068 (1981).

24. Donovan, J.J., Simon, M.I., Draper, R.K., and Montal, M. Proc. Natl. Acad. Sci. USA 78, 172 (1981).

25. Youle, R.J., and Neville, D.M., Jr. Proc. Natl. Acad. Sci. USA 77, 5483 (1980).

26. Le Bien, T.W., Bradley, J.G., and Koller, B. J. Immunol. 130, 1833 (1983).

27. Burns, G.F., Body, A.W., and Beverly, P.C.L. J. Immunol. 129, 1451 (1982).

28. Fauser, A.A. and Messner, H.A. Blood 52, 1243 (1978).

29. Ash, R.C., Detrick, R.A., and Zanjani, E.D. Blood 58, 309 (1981).

30. Vallera, D.A., Ash, R.C., Zanjani, E.D., Kersey, J.H., Le Bien, T.W., Beverly, P.C.L., Neville, D.M., Jr., and Youle, R.J. Science, in press (1983).

31. Neville, P.M., Jr. and Youle, R.J. Immunol. Revs. 62, 135 (1981).

32. Vallera, D.A., Soldering, C., Youle, R.J., Neville, D.M., Jr., and Kersey, J. Transplantation, 136 (1983).

33. Vallera, D.A., Filipovich, A., Soderling, C.C.B., and Kersey, J.H. Clin. Immunol. Path. 23, 437 (1982).

34. Bernheim, J.L. and Mendelsohn, J., in 'Regulatory Mechanism of Lymphocyte Activation', 11th Leucocyte Culture Conference (D.O. Lucas, ed.), p. 479. Academic Press, New York (1977).

35. Bondevik, H., Helgesen, A., Thoresen, A.B., and Thorsby, E. Tissue Antigens 4, 469 (1974).

36. Chang, T.M. and Kullberg, D.W. J. Biol. Chem. 257, 12563 (1982).

37. Uchida, T., Papenheimer, A.M., Jr., and Harper, A. J. Biol. Chem. 248, 3845 (1973).

38. Olsnes, S., Sandvig, K., Refsnes, K., and Pihl, A. J. Biol. Chem. 251, 3985 (1976).

39. Chang, T.M. and Neville, D.M., Jr. J. Biol. Chem. 253, 6866 (1978).

40. Heagy, W.E. and Neville, D.M., Jr. J. Biol. Chem. 256, 10618 (1981).

41. Keen, J.H., Maxfield, F.R., Hardegree, M.C., and Habig, W.H. Proc. Natl. Acad. Sci. USA 79, 2912 (1982).

42. Gottlieb, C. and Kornfeld, S. J. Biol. Chem. 251, 7761 (1976).

43. Esworthy, R.S., Youle, R.J., and Neville, D.M., Jr. Manuscript in preparation.

44. Oeltmann, T.N. and Heath, E.C. J. Biol. Chem. 254, 1028 (1979).

45. Gilliland, D.G., Steplewski, Z., Collier, R.J., Mitchell, K.F., Chang, T.H., and Koprowski, H. Proc. Natl. Acad. Sci. USA 77, 4539 (1980).

46. Cawley, D.B., Herschman, H.R., Gilliland, D.G.., and Collier, R.J. Cell 22, 563 (1980).

47. Vittetta, E.S., Krolick, K.A., Miyama-Inaba, M., Cushley, W., and Uhr, J.W. Science 219, 644 (1983).

48. Jansen, F.K., Blythman, H.D., Carriere, D., Casellas, P., Diaz, J., Gros, P., Hennequin, J.R., Taolucci, F., Tau, B., Poncelet, P., Richer, G., Salhi, S.L., Vidal, H. and Voisin, G.A. Immunol. Letts. 2, 97 (1980).

49. Thorpe, P.E., Mason, D.W., Brown, A.N.F., Simmonds, S.J., Ross, W.C.J., Cumber, A.J., and Forrester, J.A. Nature 297, 549 (1982).

50. Pappenheimer, A.M., Jr. Ann. Rev. Biochem. 46, 69 (1977).

51. Olsnes, S. and Pihl, A., in 'Receptors and Recognition, Series B' (P. Cuatrecasas, ed.), p. 129. Chapman and Hall, London (1976).

QUESTIONS AND ANSWERS

TROWBRIDGE: Are your survival curves actual survival or decay of protein synthesis?

NEVILLE: The curves are for protein synthesis decay and they correlate well with clonogenic survival assays.

MAGNANI: How did you determine that o-acetylation specifically blocked the binding site on the B subunit. Have you tried to inactivate this site with a lactose photoaffinity label?

NEVILLE: We selected conditions where acetylation was blocked by 0.5M lactose. We tried the lactose photoaffinity label and it did not work, probably because the affinity of B chain for lactose is too low. Even lactopeptides which have affinities of 10^{-5} to 10^{-7} are below the 10^{-10} affinity required for good photoaffinity labeling.

CICARELLI: Is it possible that the reduction in PHA stimulation by your anti-T cell immunotoxin is due to uptake of the toxin by accessory non-T cells (e.g., macrophages)? For example, do other immunotoxins not specific for T cells give reduced PHA responses or not?

NEVILLE: I don't know whether we have done that.

THORPE: We tried to deliberately kill macrophages by immunotoxin uptake via Fc receptors and failed despite internalization of the toxin.

VITETTA: Our experience is just the opposite. When we use control immunotoxins there is frequently a significant macrophage effect that can be reversed by adding back fresh macrophages.

BLOCKADE OF THE GALACTOSE-BINDING SITE OF RICIN BY ITS LINKAGE TO ANTIBODY

Philip Thorpe, Alex Brown, Brian Foxwell
and Christopher Myers

Imperial Cancer Research Fund
London, United Kingdom

Walter Ross, Alan Cumber and Tony Forrester

Chester Beatty Research Institute
London, United Kingdom

I. INTRODUCTION

Cell type-specific cytotoxic agents have been constructed in several laboratories by linking highly potent toxins, such as ricin, to antibody molecules (reviewed in references 1-2). Ricin, the toxin from the castor bean, is a glycoprotein composed of two polypeptide subunits, A and B, joined by a disulphide bond. The B chain binds to galactose-containing molecules that are found on the surface of most cell types, and then the A chain is believed to penetrate the cell and kill it by catalytically inactivating its ribosomes (reviewed in reference 3).

One strategy for conferring selectivity of binding upon ricin is simply to link the intact toxin directly to the antibody molecule. Conjugates of this type are powerfully cytotoxic to cells with appropriate antigens but have to be used in the presence of high concentrations of free galactose or lactose in vitro to antagonize their nonspecific binding to galactose residues on nontarget cells (4-5). The other approach that has been widely used is to couple the isolated toxin A chain directly to the antibody by a disulphide bond. Conjugates of this type, although free from the problem of nonspecific binding, show great variability in cytotoxic potency, some being as effective as the native toxin and others being only weakly cytotoxic (reviewed in 1-2).

Here we give preliminary details of a method for linking intact ricin to antibodies in a manner that produces blockade of the galactose binding properties of the toxin. Monocolonal anti-Thy1.1 antibody linked in this way to ricin was a powerful and specific cytotoxic agent, as was also a conjugate made from the W3/25 monoclonal antibody that is not cytotoxic when linked directly to ricin A chain (6-7).

II. PREPARATION OF CONJUGATES

Ricin was linked to two monoclonal antibodies, MRC OX7, specific for the Thy1.1 antigen (8), and W3/25, specific for an antigen upon thymocytes and a subset of T lymphocytes in the rat (9). The conjugation procedure was similar to that devised by Rector et al., 1978. The N-hydroxysuccinimidyl ester of iodoacetic acid was used to introduce an average of 1.5 iodoacetyl groups into each molecule of ricin (trace labeled with ^{125}I). An average of 1.7 thiol groups was incorporated into each molecule of antibody (IgG) by pyridyl-dithiolation with the SPDP reagent (Pharmacia Ltd.) and reduction with dithiothreitol. The two derivatized proteins were mixed and stirred overnight at room temperature and were then fractionated on a column of Sephadex G200. The material that eluted with a molecular weight corresponding to 210,000 (containing the simplest conjugate with one molecule of antibody linked to one of toxin) was further fractionated on acid-treated Sepharose 4B. The majority (60 to 80%) of the conjugate bound insufficiently strongly to the β-galactosyl residues of the column to be retained, whereas the remainder attached to the column and was later displaced with 0.1M galactose. A portion of the OX7-ricin conjugate that had passed through the Sepharose column was applied to an asialofetuin-Sepharose column. Only 24% of the conjugate, as detected by the radioactivity on the ricin moiety, passed through the column.

The iodoacetylated ricin intermediate was found in separate experiments to bind to Sepharose as strongly as did native ricin. Thus, the loss in Sepharose binding of the conjugate appears to be a consequence of completing the linkage of the modified ricin to the antibody. It could be that carbohydrate groups in the antibody act as affinity labels for the toxin. Alternatively, the bulky antibody moiety may sterically hinder the galactose-recognition sites of the toxin in those conjugate molecules that escaped from the columns.

III. FLUORESCENCE-ACTIVATED CELL SORTER ANALYSIS OF CELL BINDING

A fluorescence-activated cell sorter was used to analyze the specific and nonspecific binding of the OX7-ricin conjugates to cells. All fractions of the conjugate, regardless of their behavior on Sepharose and asialofetuin-Sepharose columns, bound to Thy1.1-expressing AKR mouse thymocytes and AKR-A lymphoma cells to an extent indistinguishable from that of the native antibody. When tested against Thy1.2-expressing CBA thymocytes or EL4 lymphoma cells, the conjugate that had retained Sepharose-binding capacity was observed to bind strongly, that which passed through Sepharose to bind weakly and that which passed through asialofetuin-Sepharose to show no detectable nonspecific binding even when used at 8×10^{-8}M, a concentration far in excess of that needed for saturation of antigens upon the AKR cells.

IV. CYTOTOXICITY EXPERIMENTS

All fractions of OX7-ricin were extremely powerful cytotoxic agents for AKR-A lymphoma cells in tissue culture. A one hour period of exposure of the cells to the conjugates at concentrations of $2-5 \times 10^{-12}$M reduced their capacity to incorporate ^{3}H-leucine into protein by 50% (Fig. 1). The conjugates were approximately ten times as potent as native ricin used under the same experimental conditions. When tested for nonspecific toxicity to EL4 cells, which are as sensitive to uncoupled ricin as the AKR-A cells, the OX7-ricin conjugates that passed through the Sepharose or asialofetuin-Sepharose columns were found to be toxic only at the highest concentration tested (1.5×10^{-8}M), whereas the conjugate that was retained by Sepharose exhibited marked nonspecific toxicity, reducing the leucine incorporation of the cells by half at 3×10^{-10}M. Similar results to those with the EL4 cells were

obtained using AKR-A cells coated with saturating amounts of
unconjugated OX7 antibody (results not shown).

The nonspecific toxicity of the conjugate that retained
Sepharose-binding capacity was mediated through the recognition of galactose residues on the surface of the EL4 cells and
OX7-coated AKR-A cells; this was evident from the one
hundred-fold drop in toxicity when the conjugate was applied
to these cells in the presence of 50mM lactose (results not
shown). By contrast, the weak nonspecific toxicity of the
conjugate that passed through the asialofetuin column was
antagonized little, if at all, by lactose and could possibly
have been due to fluid-phase pinocytosis of the conjugate and
proteolytic cleavage to release active ricin.

A conjugate of the monoclonal antibody W3/25 and intact
ricin was found in previous work to be highly toxic to W3/25-
expressing normal and leukemic T cells, whereas a conjugate
made with the isolated A chain was ineffective even when its
endocytosis was induced with rabbit anti-mouse immunoglobulin
antiserum (6-7). This difference suggested that the B chain
was needed directly or indirectly for the penetration of the
A chain through cell membranes into the cytosol. To investigate whether the galactose-recognition property of the B chain
was involved in the penetration process, a conjugate of W3/25
antibody and ricin was prepared and the component without
Sepharose-binding capacity purified and tested for cytotoxicity to leukemic cells. The conjugate was as potent in
its cytotoxic action as the conjugate that had retained
Sepharose-binding capacity and was ten-fold more effective
than native ricin (Fig. 2). Although not conclusive, since
the conjugate could have been cleaved intracellularly to re-
expose the galactose binding sites, this experiment provides
suggestive evidence that the property of the B chain that is
needed for the A chain to traverse cell membranes is
independent of the recognition of galactose. It could be, for

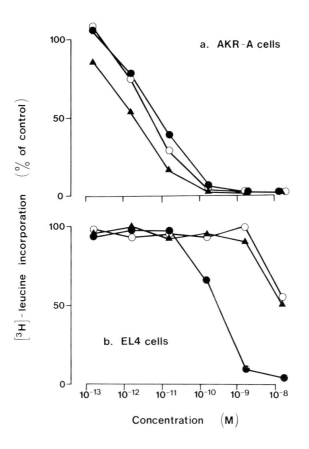

FIGURE 1. Specific and nonspecific cytotoxic effects of OX7-ricin conjugates. AKR-A (a) and EL4 (b) cells were incubated with the conjugates for 1 hr at 37°C, washed, and their capacity to incorporate ^{3}H-leucine measured 23 hr later. The conjugates tested were 1) not retained by asialofetuin-Sepharose (O), ii) not retained by Sepharose (▲) or iii) retained by Sepharose (●).

example, that hydrophobic domains on the B chain, once brought
in close contact with the cell membrane by the interaction of
the antibody moiety with antigens on the cell surface, can
complex with lipid components of the membrane with the result
that the toxin (or just its A chain) traverses the membrane by
diffusion. Ricin may thus resemble diphtheria toxin, for
which there exists compelling evidence for spontaneous
insertion into lipid membranes [both of liposomes (11) and
cells (12)] and appearance of the enzymic site of the A chain
on the far side of the membrane (11).

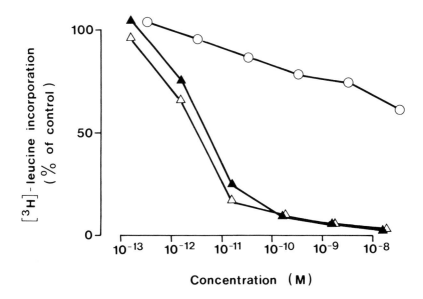

FIGURE 2. Toxic effect of W3/25 antibody conjugates upon
PVG rat leukemic cells. The cells were incubated with the
conjugates for 1h at 37°C, washed, and their capacity to
incorporate ^{3}H-leucine measured 23h later. The conjugates
tested were i) W3/25-ricin A chain (O), ii) W3/25-intact ricin
that passed through a Sepharose column (▲), or iii) W3/25-
intact ricin that was retained by a Sepharose column (Δ). The
antibody was kindly provided by Dr. D. W. Mason, Oxford.

V. CONCLUSION

The 'blocked' ricin conjugates have an advantage over intact ricin conjugates previously constructed in that they do not need to be used in the presence of high concentrations of lactose or galactose in vitro to avert nonspecific toxicity. This simplifies their use and makes more practical their application to the destruction of malignant cells in autologous marrow grafts or of T cells in allogeneic marrow grafts. They have the disadvantage when compared with A chain conjugates of greater nonspecific cytotoxicity, but this may be offset by the greater potency and consistency of the specific toxic effect that they exert. In addition, the new conjugates merit testing for therapeutic activity in vivo since, being formed with a thioether linkage, they may have better stability in animals than the disulphide—bonded A chain conjugates which are thought to be particularly prone to cleavage (13-14).

REFERENCES

1. Olsnes, S. and Pihl, A.   Pharmac. Ther. 15, 355 (1982).
2. Thorpe, P.E., Edwards, D.C., Davies, A.J.S., and Ross, W.C.J., in 'Monoclonal Antibodies in Clinical Medicine' (J. Fabre and A. McMichael, eds.), p. 167.   Academic Press, London (1982).
3. Olsnes, S. and Pihl, A., in 'Molecular Action of Toxins and Viruses' (P. Cohen and S. Van Heyningen, eds.), p. 51.   Elsevier Biomedical Press, New York (1982).
4. Youle, R.J. and Neville, D.M.   Proc. Natl. Acad. Sci. USA 77, 5483 (1980).
5. Thorpe, P.E., Cumber, A.J., Williams, N., Edwards, D.C., Ross, W.C.J., and Davies, A.J.S.   Clin. Exp. Immunol. 43, 195 (1981).
6. Thorpe, P.E. and Ross, W.C.J.   Immunol. Reviews 62, 119 (1982).
7. Mason, D.W., Thorpe, P.E., and Ross, W.C.J.   Cancer Surveys 1, 389 (1982).
8. Mason, D.W. and Williams, A.F.   Biochem. J. 187, 1 (1980).
9. Brideau, R.J., Carter, P.B., McMaster, W.R., Mason, D.W., and Williams, A.F.   Eur. J. Immunol. 10, 609 (1980).
10. Rector, E.S., Schwenk, R.J., Tse, K.S., and Sehon, A.H. J. Immunol. Methods 24, 321 (1978).

11. Donovan, J., Simon, M., and Montal, M.   Biophys. J. 37, 256a (1982).
12. Sandvig, K. and Olsnes, S.   J. Biol. Chem. 256, 9068 (1981).
13. Edwards, D.C., Ross, W.C.J., Cumber, A.J., McIntosh, D., Smith, A., Thorpe, P.E., Brown, A., Williams, R.H., and Davies, A.J.S.   Biochim. Biophys. Acta 717, 272 (1982).
14. Jansen, F.K., Blythman, H.E., Carrière, D., Casellas, P., Gros, O., Gros, P., Laurent, J.C., Paolucci, F., Pau, B. and Poncelet, P.   Immunol. Rev. 62, 185 (1982).

QUESTIONS AND ANSWERS

NEVILLE: Have you looked at the kinetics of protein synthesis inactivation with your 'blocked' conjugate? How long does it take to reduce protein synthesis to 0.01% of control?

THORPE: Yes, the rates of kill of 'blocked' and 'unblocked' ricin conjugates are identical in the presence of lactose, and this is slightly less than for the native ricin.

TROWBRIDGE: Have the ricin-resistant cell lines which lack binding sites been tested as targets for B chain-containing immunotoxins to see if the B chain is doing something more than simply promoting binding?

THORPE: Not to my knowledge. It would be very interesting to look at this with cell lines defective in ricin transport as well.

MONOCLONAL ANTIBODY CONJUGATES FOR DIAGNOSTIC IMAGING AND THERAPY

Mette Strand[1]
David A. Scheinberg[2]

The Johns Hopkins University School of Medicine
Department of Pharmacology and
Experimental Therapeutics
Baltimore, Maryland

Otto A. Gansow[1]

Michigan State University
Department of Chemistry
East Lansing, Michigan

A. M. Friedman[1]

Argonne National Laboratory, Chemistry Division
Argonne, Illinois

I. INTRODUCTION

We have used a murine tumor system as a model to study the diagnostic and therapeutic potential of monoclonal antibody conjugates as drugs. The pharmacological principles of these studies should be applicable to monoclonal antibody diagnosis and therapy in humans, even though the absolute quantitative values may differ among the many neoplastic diseases encountered.   The system is the Rauscher leukemia virus-induced erythroblastic leukemia of mice.

---

[1]This work supported by NCI-N01CP81052
[2]DAS supported by MSTP GM07309

The monoclonal antibody designated 103A, an IgG1, was specific for the Rauscher leukemia virus envelope glycoprotein gp 70, which is expressed in large amounts on the cell surface of the leukemia cells (1). Controls included the P3 immuno-globulin, produced by P3Ag8 myeloma cells (2), and 263D (both class IgG1).

The 103A IgG specifically bound to the leukemia cells and did not react with normal cells, whereas the control immuno-globulins did not bind to any of these cells (1). Uptake ratios of the specific immunoglobulin or its $F(ab')_2$ fragments on tumor cells as compared to normal cells in live animals were more than 60-fold greater (1). Kinetic analysis of targeting indicated maximal tumor targeting occurred in six hours or less, with subsequent rapid loss of antibody from the tumor (3). The specific targeting and high uptake ratios thus allowed us to conduct both diagnostic imaging and therapeutic studies in this system.

II. IMAGING

A number of radiohalides and radiometals may be conjugated to monoclonal antibodies for diagnostic imaging (discussed in 3). The most versatile method of radiolabeling of anti-bodies for imaging was the use of bifunctional radiometal chelates. These chelates can bind indium 111, gallium 67, and technetium 99m, all short-lived γ emitters of suitable energy (4-7). Of these, the bifunctional chelates prepared with diethylenetriaminepentaacetic acid appeared to be the most useful because of the ease of conjugation and their retention of biological activity and stability in vivo (5,8). High resolution images of tumors can be obtained using the radio-metal chelate-conjugated specific antibody (5). Direct comparisons showed these images to be far superior to those obtained using ^{131}I-labeled monoclonal immunoglobulins (3).

The kinetics of antibody targeting and catabolism were studied using mice injected with ^{125}I-labeled antibody and papain digestion fragments. In leukemic mice, where a target existed, there was a direct correlation between the specific uptake of iodine in the spleen and the accumulation of iodine in the stomach, thus indicating that specific catabolism of the targeted antibody had occurred (3). In addition, it appeared that: 1) the catabolism of the tumor-bound antibody occurred very rapidly (we observed a 5- to 7-fold loss of antibody from the spleen in 18 hours); 2) the problem of specific catabolism of bound antibody appeared to be

independent of immunoglobulin class or fragment; and
3) tumor-bound antibody was rapidly cleared from the blood as
it bound to antigen. Likewise, studies using radiometal
chelate-conjugated monoclonal antibodies showed that specific
targeting resulted in catabolism and subsequent accumulation
of radioactivity in organs metabolizing metals (3).

III. THERAPY

The therapeutic effects of the tumor-specific monoclonal
antibody against the Rauscher erythroleukemia were also
assessed (1). A dose-response relationship between antibody
103A and inhibition of both tumor foci and splenomegaly was
obtained; the 50% effective dose at blocking tumor growth was
1.5 μg. We have used this dose-response curve as a baseline
for quantitative measurement of the therapeutic effects of
cytocidal agents conjugated to monoclonal antibodies. Several
possible agents are listed (Table 1) (discussed in 8).

TABLE 1. Cytotoxic Agents

Halides	Drugs	Biologically Active Molecules
iodine 131	methotrexate	RNAse
iodine 125	α-amanitin	phospholipase
bromine 77	daunomycin	cobra venom factor

Protein Toxins	Liposomes
diphtheria A chain	(containing many
ricin A chain	substances)
abrin	
gelonin	Bifunctional
other bacterial toxins	Chelates and
	Cryptates
	scandium 47
	bismuth 212
	actinides

Iodine 131 is the simplest agent to attach and the one that has been used most extensively (9). In our system, however, ^{131}I-labeled antibody was no more potent than the unlabeled antibody in vivo. This lack of potency may result from the long-range emission characteristics of ^{131}I and its eight day half-life as compared to a seven hour half-life of the ^{131}I-103A IgG on the tumor cells (1).

Methotrexate-IgG and diphtheria A chain-IgG conjugates were also examined. Methotrexate-IgG conjugates were less potent than free methotrexate in vitro and lost specificity of binding (8). The toxin-conjugated antibodies did not appear useful because the disulfide linkage was labile in vivo (10). However, successful application of these types of conjugates are reviewed elsewhere in this volume.

Other highly cytotoxic agents are the α-emitting isotopes, such as bismuth 212, which can be conjugated to the chelated, derivatized IgG as described above for indium (3,5). This isotope has the advantages of much greater tumoricidal effects due to extremely large linear energy transfer (LET) and reduced possibility of damaging normal cells in the vicinity of the tumor due to the 40–90μm range of the emitted particles. For example, if ^{212}Bi had been substituted for ^{111}In in our previous experiments (5), several thousand rads of high LET radiation would have been delivered to the leukemic spleen, a dose far in excess of that required to kill every leukemic cell.

Cell killing by radiolabeled antibodies in vitro was investigated to approximate their therapeutic potency. Iodine 125–, iodine 131–, bismuth 212–labeled antibodies and unlabeled antibody were added to leukemia cells and incubated for various times. Surviving cells were enumerated using a Coulter counter (Figure 1).

Unlabeled and ^{125}I-labeled antibody were not cytotoxic, even at very high concentrations. ^{131}I-103A IgG was able to kill cells at high doses, but killing depended on the length of time the radiolabeled IgG was incubated with the cells. As noted earlier, in live animals the radioiodine has a very short half-life at the tumor cell surface, suggesting that the killing observed in vitro will greatly exceed the killing in vivo. We have observed no killing by targeted iodine 131 in our in vivo system (see above). On the other hand, ^{212}Bi-103A IgG was extremely potent, despite its low specific activity in these experiments and the one hour half-life of the isotope.

Unfortunately, there was equally potent killing by the radiolabeled control IgGs. In the case of iodine 131, due to the long pathlength of the β particles there was sufficient radiation in the media above the cells to account for non-

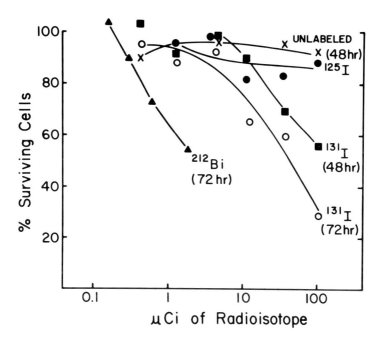

FIGURE 1.   Cell killing by radiolabeled 103A IgG in vitro.
Dilutions of unlabeled or labeled IgG were added to 10^5 F46
leukemia cells in 1ml media in $2cm^2$ tissue culture wells. The
cells were incubated 48 or 72 hours as indicated, and then the
percentage of surviving cells determined. ▲, ^{212}Bi-103A IgG.
O, ^{131}I-103A IgG. ■ , ^{131}I-103A IgG. ●, ^{125}I-103A IgG.
X, unlabeled 103A IgG.   The unlabeled IgG was added at the
same concentration as used in the iodine experiments: 10μg/ml
in the lowest dilution. Specific activities: ^{125}I and ^{131}I,
10μCi/μg; ^{212}Bi, 0.1μCi/μg.

specific killing. In the case of the bismuth 212, limitations
in the specific activity of the IgG and consequent large
amounts of IgG in close association with the cells within the
geometry of the wells resulted in high nonspecific
cytotoxicity.   However, despite these problems in vitro,
bismuth 212 remains the most potent isotope for conjugation.
     Initial experiments have been carried out to investigate
the biodistribution and stability of chelated radioactive
bismuth.   As expected, the bismuth was retained within the
chelate and very rapidly cleared through the kidneys, with no

significant organ uptake. In contrast, injections of radioactive bismuth as free metal resulted in more than 16 percent
retention of the injected dose 18 hours after injection (10).
Experiments assessing the specificity and potency of
^{212}Bi-103A IgG in vivo are in progress.

IV.   CONCLUSIONS

A.   Targeting to tumor cells was rapid.   In the leukemic
model described here, binding occurred almost immediately.
B.   Specific targeting or binding of monoclonal antibody
resulted in an extremely rapid loss of the antibody from the
vasculature.
C.   The specifically bound antibody (but not unbound antibody) was rapidly catabolized, resulting in radioactivity in
excretory organs such as the stomach (when iodinated antibody
was used) or in tissues that metabolize metals such as the
liver (when radiometal-conjugated immunoglobulins were used).
D.   Optimal imaging was obtained immediately after extravascular distribution of the antibody; therefore, regardless
of the system, short-lived isotopes such as iodine 123,
technetium 99m, gallium 68, or indium 111 will be
advantageous.
E.   Monoclonal IgG could be used alone as an antineoplastic drug with reproducible pharmacokinetics and dose-
response characteristics.   However, underivatized antibody may
not be successful in humans with significant tumor or antigen
loads, and conjugates of antibodies with extremely potent
cytotoxic agents will probably be necessary in these cases.
F.   Antibody conjugated to iodine 131, iodine 125,
antineoplastic drugs or protein toxins was not useful in this
system.   Radiometal conjugates containing potent, short-lived
α emitters such as bismuth 212 may be most useful.

ACKNOWLEDGMENTS

We thank W. Anderson for help with the bifunctional
chelate experiments and Ms. L. Poole for typing the
manuscript.

ABBREVIATIONS

LET, linear energy transfer.

REFERENCES

1. Scheinberg, D.A. and Strand, M. Cancer Res. 42, 44 (1982).
2. Kohler, G., Howe, S.C., and Milstein, C. Eur. J. Immunol. 6, 292 (1976).
3. Scheinberg, D. A. and Strand, M. Cancer Res. 43, 265 (1983).
4. Scheinberg, D. A., Strand, M., and Gansow, O., in 'Monoclonal Antibodies in Drug Development', (J. T. August, ed.) Am. Soc. for Pharmacology and Experimental Therapeutics, Bethesda, Maryland (1981).
5. Scheinberg, D. A., Strand, M., and Gansow, O. Science 215, 1511 (1982).
6. Khaw, B.A., Fallon, J.T., Strauss, H.W., and Haber, E. Science 209, 295 (1980).
7. Khaw, B..A., Strauss, W., Carvalho, A., Locke, E., Gold, H.K., and Haber, E. J. Nucl. Med. 23, 1011 (1982).
8. Scheinberg, D. A., Anderson, W. and Strand, M., in 'Radioimmunoimaging' (S. Burchiel and B. Rhodes, eds.). Elsevier, New York (1983).
9. Goldenberg, D.M. Cancer Res. 40, 2953 (1980).
10. Strand, M., Scheinberg, D. A., and Gansow, O., in 'Cell Fusion: Gene Transfer and Transformation' (Miles International Symposium #14) (R.F. Beers and E.G. Bassett, eds.) p 385. Raven Press, New York (1983).

QUESTIONS AND ANSWERS

THORPE: You said that the in vivo half-life of ricin antibody conjugates was very short and therefore you discontinued using them. I wonder how you measured the half-life.

STRAND: We iodinated the ricin and diphtheria toxin A chain conjugate. We injected this into animals intraveneously or intraperitoneally and took serum samples at hourly intervals for 24 hours. Samples were then run on gels and assayed for the position of radioactivity. In both cases within five hours the toxin was no longer associated with the antibody.

Human Monoclonal Antibodies

CONSTRUCTION OF HETEROMYELOMAS FOR HUMAN MONOCLONAL ANTIBODY PRODUCTION

Nelson N. H. Teng, Francisco Calvo-Riera,
Kit S. Lam, and Henry S. Kaplan

Cancer Biology Research Laboratory
Department of Radiology
Stanford University School of Medicine
Stanford, California

I. INTRODUCTION

The development by Köhler and Milstein (1) of the mouse-mouse hybridoma procedure for mouse monoclonal antibody production has opened a new era in immunology. The fact that the cloned hybridoma cell lines thus derived are immortal assures permanent availability of their antibody products, and antibody titer in these cases is limited only by cell culture volume. However, clinical use of xenoantibodies in human patients is likely to be severely limited by the fact that they will be treated as foreign proteins by the human immune system. Accordingly, for diagnostic and therapeutic applications in man, the production of human (rather than mouse or other rodent) monoclonal antibodies through appropriate modifications of the hybridoma procedure would clearly be desirable.

The first attempts to generate immortalized human immunoglobulin-producing cells involved the fusion of human lymphoid cells with mouse myeloma cells to create chimeric hybridomas (2,3,4). However, with rare exceptions (5,6), such mouse-human hybridomas have tended to be unstable and to cease human immunoglobulin production due to the selective loss of human chromosomes (7,8) or to disturbances of gene expression (9). A second approach involved the transformation of antigen-primed human B lymphocytes with the Epstein-Barr virus (EBV) (10,11,12); this method has had some success, but

appears to be of limited practical usefulness because such
cultures have tended to cease antibody production after a
variable period (10). Still more recently, several groups
have succeeded in fusing mutant human myeloma cell lines with
antigen-primed human B lymphocytes to yield human-human
hybridomas secreting monoclonal antibodies of predefined
antigenic specificity (13,14,15). However, only a few human
myeloma cell lines have been permanently established in
culture, and essentially all of these are relatively slow
growing and therefore vulnerable to suppression of the
malignant phenotype (16,17) after fusion with antigen-primed
normal human B lymphocytes, resulting in an undesirably low
yield of viable hybridomas. Accordingly, there is an urgent
need for the development of new malignant fusion partner cell
lines capable of generating high yields of viable hybridomas
and high, sustained levels of human monoclonal antibody
production following fusion with antigen-primed human
B lymphocytes. This paper presents a preliminary report of
the construction of novel mouse-human hybrid myeloma (heteromyeloma) cell lines which appear to have significantly more
favorable characteristics as malignant fusion partners for the
production of human monoclonal antibodies.

II. MATERIALS AND METHODS

Details of technical procedures will be published
elsewhere. Briefly, a new hypoxanthine-aminopterin-
thymidine(HAT)-sensitive mutant of the U-266 human myeloma
cell line (18) was derived by selection of the cells in
6-thioguanine (6-TG) after first freeing the parental myeloma
cells (kindly provided by Dr. Nilsson, Uppsala, Sweden) of
mycoplasma infection by heat treatment at $41^{\circ}C$ for 44 hours.
The 6-TG-resistant cells were shown to be HAT sensitive;
unlike an earlier mutant, U-266 AR_1 (SKO-007), derived by
selection in 8-azaguanine (14), they revealed no detectable
level of leakiness or reversion in HAT medium. Like the
parental U-266 cell line, FU-266 cells have a modal number of
44 chromosomes, secrete IgE (λ), and have a doubling time of
approximately 40-45 hours. Their capacity to act as malignant
fusion partners in fusions with antigen-primed human B lymphocytes is poor, and similar or inferior to that of the
previously described SKO-007 mutant (13).
        The next step involved the transfection into FU-266 cells
of a bacterial gene for neomycin resistance, using a
recombinant plasmid vector, pSV-2 neo^r, constructed by Dr.
Paul Berg and co-workers in the Department of Biochemistry,

Stanford University School of Medicine (19). The protoplast fusion technique (20) was used, with minor modifications, and the transfected myeloma cells were then incubated in the presence of the antibiotic G-418 (Schering Corporation). Viable growth occurred in several culture wells; each of these cultures was cloned and expanded, and growth curves were determined. The fastest growing clone, designated E-1, was selected for further study. There was no detectable alteration in the biological properties of the transfected E-1 cells with respect to HAT sensitivity, IgE (λ) secretion, growth rate, or capacity to yield human-human hybridomas.

The P3X63Ag.8.653-NP HAT-sensitive mouse myeloma cell line (21) was selected as the murine malignant fusion partner because of its rapid growth rate, excellent fusion characteristics, and loss of the capacity to secrete mouse immunoglobulin. This cell line was incubated in the presence of the antibiotic G-418 and found to be highly sensitive, with no survivors after approximately ten days. Two sets of fusions of FU-266 (clone E-1) x P3X63Ag.8.653-NP cells were carried out, using a previously described procedure (22) with minor modifications (23). Since it is well established that human cells are significantly more sensitive to ouabain than mouse cells, selection of the fused heteromyelomas was then carried out in the presence of ouabain plus G-418. In the first series of fusions, in which intact, unirradiated mouse myeloma cells were used, approximately 30 hybrid clones were obtained of which a small number (A-6, A-10, B-6) were selected for further study. The second series of fusions was carried out after exposing the mouse myeloma cells to a single sublethal dose of gamma irradiation, which was intended to damage some of the murine chromosomes and thus favor the retention of an increased number of human chromosomes (24). Selection was again carried out in the presence of ouabain plus G-418. Once again, many clones were obtained, of which a small number (D36, D3, D33) were selected for further study.

Several test fusions with polyclonally activated human B lymphocytes, with antigen-primed human B lymphocytes, and with an uncloned line, C-10, of anti-tetanus toxoid antibody-producing, EBV-transformed human lymphoblastoid cells have been performed. The initial fusions were carried out with individual heteromyeloma clones, usually in comparison with the murine or human parental myeloma. More recently, large scale comparison fusions have been carried out with several of these heteromyelomas, and with the parental mouse myeloma, using the same preparations of human B lymphocytes as the normal fusion partner for all of the tested malignant fusion partner cells. These fusions were carried out with pokeweed mitogen-stimulated peripheral blood lymphocytes (PWM-PBL), with normal human spleen B lymphocytes, and with the C-10 human lymphoblastoid cell line, again using a standard polyethylene glycol fusion procedure (22) with minor modifications (23). Selection following all of these fusions was carried out in HAT medium (25). Secretion of human IgM and/or IgG was determined by the enzyme-linked immunosorbent assay (ELISA) (26).

III. RESULTS

The heteromyelomas obtained following fusion of clone E-1 with unirradiated P3X63Ag.8.653-NP mouse myeloma cells, of which A-6 and A-10 are prototype clones, had doubling times ranging from 15-22 hours. The ouabain sensitivities of the heteromyelomas varied considerably; those most sensitive to ouabain were only slightly more resistant than human cells, whereas those most insensitive, including A-6, were about as resistant as the parental mouse myeloma. As expected, all of the heteromyelomas remained HAT sensitive, since both parental cells were HAT sensitive and selection was carried out in the absence of HAT. Chromosome analysis verified that these heteromyelomas were human-mouse somatic cell hybrids containing variable total numbers of chromosomes, ranging from 50-110; only one human chromosome was present in most of the hybrids, but some contained up to three human chromosomes. Clone A-6 had a total of 98 chromosomes of which two and a possible third were human. Surface membrane and cytoplasmic immunofluorescence studies, using heterologous antibodies prepared against the FU-266 human myeloma cell line, demonstrated the presence of human antigens in most of the heteromyelomas. Similar observations were made with the heteromyeloma clones obtained after fusion of irradiated P3X63Ag.8.653-NP cells with clone E-1. Chromosome analysis revealed that these hybrids tended to retain a greater number of human chromosomes, ranging from 3-8 per clone. Clone D36, which was one of the most rapidly growing, contained a total of 93 chromosomes, of which five were definitely human in morphology. Although all of the heteromyeloma clones initially produced IgE (λ), most became nonproducers after a few weeks in culture. Like the first series of clones, they were HAT sensitive and resistant to both ouabain and G-418. Certain of the heteromyeloma clones have been consistently superior to others, and to the parental mouse myeloma cell line, in test fusions with human B lymphocytes. Of these, clone D36 from the second set of heteromyeloma fusions and clone A-6 from the first set of such fusions appear to be outstanding. However, other heteromyelomas have also yielded

good results in isolated fusions. Thus, a fusion of heteromyeloma clone A-10 with PWM-PBL yielded fifteen human immunoglobulin-secreting hybridomas which have been tested at serial
intervals and have remained stable producers for about six
months. In another fusion involving heteromyeloma A-6 and the
uncloned C-10 human lymphoblastoid cell line, a hybridoma
designated #77 has produced specific IgM (κ) monoclonal antibody against tetanus toxoid for over five months. Biosyn-
thetic radiolabeling of this clone with ^{14}C-leucine revealed
the presence of monoclonal human μ and κ chains in autoradio-
grams of polyacrylamide electrophoresis gels. More recent
fusions involving heteromyeloma clone D36 with PWM-PBL and
with the anti-tetanus toxoid antibody-producing human lymphoblastoid line C-10 have yielded an approximately 100%
incidence of viable hybridomas. Over 90% of the wells
containing viable hybridomas were shown by ELISA assays to be
producing human IgM and/or IgG. The levels of immunoglobulin
secretion have not yet been determined precisely, but rough
estimates based on comparison with IgM and IgG standards in
the ELISA test plates suggest that many hybridoma clones are
producing between 10 and 50µg/ml. As expected from the fact
that the parental heteromyeloma clones are nonproducers, these
hybridoma supernatants contained no detectable mouse immunoglobulin or human epsilon heavy chain. Moreover, no evidence
of permuted immunoblobulin molecules was observed in biosyn-
thetically labeled supernatant culture fluids analyzed by
polyacrylamide gel electrophoresis.

IV. DISCUSSION

There are many important clinical applications for which
human monoclonal antibodies would be highly desirable (27).
However, the few human myeloma cell lines in existence have
proven to be clearly less than satisfactory as malignant
fusion partners. In contrast, perhaps in part because there
have been so many murine myeloma cell lines to choose from,
several mutant mouse myeloma cell lines are now available
which are remarkably efficient and reliable as malignant
fusion partners in mouse-mouse hybridoma production. Unfortunately, when these mouse myeloma cell lines are fused with
antigen-primed human B lymphocytes, the capacity of the
resultant mouse-human hybridomas to secrete human monoclonal
antibody is usually transient due to the selective, often
rapid, elimination of human chromosomes (7,8).
        Accordingly, we have devised a strategy aimed at retaining
the outstanding fusion characteristics of the HAT-sensitive

mouse myeloma cell line P3X63Ag.8.653-NP (21) under selection
conditions in which it is forced to retain at least one human
chromosome bearing a bacterial gene for neomycin resistance
introduced by the protoplast fusion procedure. It was hoped
that, in at least some of the novel 'heteromyelomas' thus
constructed, there would be a significant decrease in the
propensity for the loss of additional human chromosomes
introduced during secondary fusions with normal human
B lymphocytes, thus providing a higher yield of viable mouse-
human hybridomas capable of stable human immunoglobulin
secretion. This approach had two further advantages. The
heteromyeloma progeny, like the parental mouse and human
myeloma cell lines, remained HAT sensitive, since selection
was carried out in ouabain and G-418; thus, the tedious step
of reselecting HAT sensitive mutants of these hybrids in
6-thioguanine or 8-azaguanine was obviated. Secondly, the
mouse myeloma cell line used had previously been selected as a
nonproducer, and it was therefore expected that its heteromyeloma progeny would also be incapable of secreting mouse
immunoglobulins. Only small numbers of human chromosomes
derived from the IgE (λ)-secreting human myeloma parent were
retained in the heteromyelomas, and most of them must have
lost human chromosomes 14 and 22, since they soon stopped
secreting human myeloma IgE (λ). Accordingly, the immunoglobulins secreted by hybridomas resulting from the fusion of
these heteromyeloma clones with antigen-primed human B lymphocytes are not diluted by the presence of other immunoglobulin
molecules, and no permuted immunoglobulin molecules appear to
be present in the culture supernatant fluids.
   The high yield of viable hybridomas, their capacity for
sustained secretion of relatively high levels of immunoglobulin, and the absence of permuted immunoglobulin molecules
in the culture supernatants strongly suggest that these
heteromyeloma clones are likely to prove uniquely favorable as
malignant fusion partners for human monoclonal antibody
production. Additional studies are now in progress to further
define which of the heteromyeloma clones works best under
various experimental conditions. When these ongoing studies
have been completed, it is anticipated that these heteromyeloma clones will be made available to interested scientists
for investigative purposes.

ABBREVIATIONS

   EBV, Epstein-Barr virus; HAT, hypoxanthine-aminopterin-
thymidine; 6-TG, 6-thioguanine; PWM-PBL, pokeweed mitogen-

stimulated peripheral blood lymphocytes; ELISA, enzyme-linked
immunosorbent assay.

REFERENCES

1. Kohler, G. and Milstein, C.   Nature 256, 495 (1975).
2. Schwaber, J. and Cohen, E.P.   Nature 244, 444 (1973).
3. Schwaber, J.   Exp. Cell Res. 93, 343 (1975).
4. Levy, R. and Dilley, J.   Proc. Natl. Acad. Sci. USA 75,
   2411 (1978).
5. Schlom, J., Wunderlich, D. and Teramoto, Y.A.   Proc.
   Natl. Acad. Sci. USA 77, 6841 (1980).
6. Lane, H.C., Shelhamer, J.H., Mostowski, H.S.. and
   Fauci, A.S.   J. Exp. Med. 155, 333 (1982).
7. Weiss, M.C. and Green, H..   Proc. Natl. Acad. Sci. USA
   58, 1104 (1967).
8. Nabholz, M., Miggiano, V. and Bodmer, W.   Nature 223, 358
   (1969).
9. Raison, R.L., Walker, K.Z., Halnan, C.R.E., Briscoe, D.
   and Basten, A.   J. Exp. Med 156, 1380 (1982).
10. Zurawski, V.R., Jr., Haber, E., and Black, P.H.   Science
    199, 1439 (1978).
11. Steinitz, M., Seppala, I., Eichmann, K., and Klein, G.
    Immunobiology 156, 44 (1979).
12. Kozbor, D., Steinitz, M., Klein, G., Koskimies, S., and
    Makela, O.   Scand. J. Immunol. 10, 187 (1979).
13. Olsson, L. and Kaplan, H.S.   Proc. Natl. Acad. Sci. USA
    77, 5429 (1980).
14. Croce, C.M., Linnenbach, A., Hall, W., Steplewski, Z.,
    and Koprowski, H.   Nature 288, 488 (1980).
15. Sikora, K., Alderson, T., Phillips, J., and Watson, J.V.
    Lancet, January 2, 11 (1982).
16. Harris, H., Miller, O.J., Klein, G., Worst, P. and
    Tachibana, T.   Nature 223, 363 (1969).
17. Stanbridge, E.J.   Nature 260, 17 (1976).
18. Nilsson, K., Bennich, H., Johansson, S.G.O., and
    Ponten, J.   Clin. Exp. Immunol. 7, 477 (1970).
19. Southern, P.J. and Berg, P.   J. of Mol. and Applied Gen.
    1, 327 (1982).
20. Shaffner, W.   Proc. Natl. Acad. Sci. USA 77, 2163 (1980).
21. Kearney, J.F., Radbruch, A., Liesegang, B., and
    Rajewsky, K.   J. Immunol. 123, 1548 (1979).
22. Oi, V.T. and Herzenberg, L.A., in 'Selected Methods in
    Cellular Immunology' (B.B. Mishell and S.M. Shiigi,
    eds.), p. 351.   W.H. Freeman Pub., San Francisco (1979).
23. Schneiderman, S., Farber, J.L., and Baserga, R.   Somatic
    Cell Genetics 5, 263 (1979).

24. Pontecorvo, G. Nature 230, 367 (1971).
25. Littlefield, J.W. Science 145, 709 (1964).
26. Engvall, E. Med. Biol. 55, 193 (1977).
27. Kaplan, H.S., Olsson, L., and Raubitschek, A., in 'Monoclonal Antibodies in Clinical Medicine' (A. McMichael and J. Fabre, eds.), p. 17. Academic Press, London (1982).

QUESTIONS AND ANSWERS

LEVY: In retrospect, was it necessary to introduce the neomycin-resistance plasmid now that you have shown that the irradiation of the mouse line works well?

KAPLAN: I suppose not, but we wasted a lot of time determining the right radiation dose and it is still very much quicker to transfect in the dominant drug marker. Furthermore, selecting for ouabain resistance, etc., is rather tedious compared with HAT markers or transfection.

HUMAN HYBRIDOMAS: COMPARISON OF HUMAN CELL LINES FOR PRODUCTION OF HUMAN HYBRIDOMAS AND DEVELOPMENT OF HUMAN HYBRIDOMAS PRODUCING ANTIGEN-SPECIFIC IgG USING IN VITRO-IMMUNIZED PERIPHERAL BLOOD CELLS AS FUSING PARTNERS[1]

Kenneth A. Foon, Paul G. Abrams, Jeffrey L. Rossio,
James A. Knost, and Robert K. Oldham

Biological Therapeutics Branch
Biological Response Modifiers Program
Division of Cancer Treatment
National Cancer Institute
Frederick Cancer Research Facility
Frederick, Maryland

I. INTRODUCTION

In nearly simultaneous achievements, Croce et al. (1) and Olsson and Kaplan (2) suggested that human-human hybridomas might follow a pattern similar to that of murine monoclonal antibodies as first reported by Köhler and Milstein (3). Unfortunately, human hybridomas have been extremely difficult to develop due to inadequacies of both of the partners required for fusion: the available human myeloma lines have been disappointing in comparison with their murine counterparts, and human B lymphocytes producing specific immunoglobulin represent a very small percentage of circulating lymphocytes or lymph node cells as compared with the splenocytes of a hyperimmunized mouse. We decided to address both of these problems by first comparing the available human lines for their utility in forming stable, immunoglobulin-secreting hybrids, and second, determining if in vitro-sensitized human

[1]Supported in part by a DHHS Grant under contract number N01-CO-23910 with Program Resources, Inc.

lymphocytes could be used as fusion partners to develop human hybridomas.

The first part of this experiment was to compare the available human myeloma and B lymphoblastoid lines. We required a 'standard' human B lymphocyte as the fusion partner which could be easily obtained in large quantities and was not dependent on donor response to a specific antigen. Hatzubai and co-workers (4) had demonstrated that secretion of the monoclonal immunoglobulin expressed on the cell surface of human B lymphoma cells could be achieved by fusion of these cells to murine myeloma NS-1. We identified a patient with an IgMk chronic lymphocytic leukemia (CLL) whose peripheral blood leukemia cells were chosen as a fusing partner for the comparison of the human lines because:

i) an abundant and continuing supply of cells was easily obtained without requiring immunization or in vitro sensitization;

ii) 99% of these cells were B cells of clonal origin and all of the CLL cells should have had comparable ability to produce immunoglobulin-secreting hybridomas;

iii) except for UC729-6, which secreted IgM at low levels that could have been subtracted for purposes of identifying positive wells, none of the human lines secreted IgM, so that testing of the hybrids for secretion could have been easily performed with an enzyme-linked immunosorbent assay (ELISA) designed to detect human IgM;

iv) in separate experiments we failed to transform these particular CLL cells with Epstein-Barr virus (EBV), so that any growth in the wells could have been ascribed to hybrid formation and not to infection of lymphocytes by EBV from virus-positive human cell lines;

v) these particular cells were previously demonstrated to form hybrids with both murine and human myeloma cells and to secrete the surface membrane IgMk.

This system provides a basis for choosing the best cell line of those tested for use in human-human hybridoma studies. In addition, it determines the most promising cell lines to use for the induction of idiotype secretion from human lymphoma and leukemia cells, and thus may have a role in the treatment of these diseases (5).

In a second set of experiments we wanted to determine if we could fuse in vitro-sensitized human lymphocytes to a human myeloma cell line to develop an antibody-secreting human hybridoma. Following the techniques of Lane et al. (6) and Misiti and Waldmann (7) for in vitro sensitization (with soluble antigens) of lymphocytes from human peripheral blood, we applied these methods to generate specifically sensitized cells for use in human-human fusions.

II. MATERIALS AND METHODS

A. Cell Lines

Human cell lines were maintained in Roswell Park Memorial Institute medium 1640 (RPMI 1640) supplemented with sodium pyruvate (1mM), L-glutamine (2mM) and 15% fetal calf serum which was supplemented with either 8-azaguanine or 6-thioguanine (both at 10^{-4}M) (Table 1). U-266 and RPMI 8226 were found to be free of mycoplasma and were selected in increasing concentrations of 8-azaguanine until a mutant sensitive to aminopterin was established. The cells were maintained in RPMI medium plus 15% fetal calf serum and 8-azaguanine (10^{-4}M). These mutants were both developed in this laboratory. UC729-6, HF_2 (a clone of UC729-6), HMy_2, and GM4672 were the other human cell lines supplied for these experiments and were grown according to suppliers' instructions.

B. Fusions and Cloning

Fifty milliliters of blood, obtained from a patient with CLL and demonstrated by flow cytometry to have surface membrane IgMk, were isolated on a Ficoll-Hypaque gradient and washed twice with serum-free RPMI 1640 medium. Fusions were performed as previously described using 10^8 CLL cells with 10^7 cells from each cell line and polyethylene glycol 1000 (8). Three fusions, each by a different investigator, were performed with each human cell line.

C. Screening for IgM Production

Ninety-six well soft vinyl plates were coated with goat anti-human Ig and negative controls, parent cell line supernatants, and a positive control human IgM were added to different wells. After one hour of incubation at room temperature, an alkaline phosphatase-conjugated goat anti-human mu chain (Sigma) was added to each well. After another hour incubation at room temperature, p-nitrophenylphosphate was added to the wells and incubated for exactly thirty minutes at room temperature. Optical densities were read at 405λ on a microELISA reader. Assay details have been described (8).

TABLE 1. Characteristics of Human Cell Line Mutants

Designation	Immunoglobulin Secreted	Source
U-266 (Myeloma)	IgE	BRMP-NCI*
RPMI 8226 (Myeloma)	Lambda light chain	BRMP-NCI*
UC729-6 (B lymphoblastoid)	IgM	Univ. of Calif. San Diego
UC729-HF$_2$ (B lymphoblastoid) (HF$_2$)	Nonsecretor	Techniclone, Inc.
LICR-LON-HMy$_2$ (B lymphoblastoid) (HMy$_2$)	IgG	Ludwig Institute for Cancer Res.
GM4672 (B lymphoblastoid)	IgG	Wistar Institute

* Biological Response Modifiers Program – National Cancer Institute

D. Culture Conditions for In Vitro Sensitization With Tetanus Toxoid

Normal individuals previously immunized with tetanus toxoid were used as donors. Mononuclear cells were isolated on Ficoll-Hypaque and the antigen used was soluble tetanus toxoid (Lederle, Pearl River, NY). Details of this in vitro system have been previously reported (9).

E. Assay for Antibody

Antibody production was tested using an enzyme-linked immunosorbent assay (ELISA), as described by Lane et al. (6).

F. Hybridoma Production

In vitro-sensitized lymphocytes were collected from six wells of a twenty-four well plate after 6, 7, 8, 9 and 10 days of in vitro exposure to tetanus toxoid. These cells were fused with an equal number of cells from a hypoxanthine-aminopterin-thymidine-sensitive subline of the human myeloma cell line U266 that was produced in our laboratories.

On day 30, extensive cell growth was seen in each of the twenty-four wells from all five plates (days 6-10 of in vitro incubation). Supernatant samples of 0.15ml were taken for testing in the ELISA, and positive wells were cloned, retested, and recloned.

III. RESULTS

A. Comparison of Human Cell Lines

The combined results of three separate fusions with the six human cell lines and one fusion with the NS-1 murine line are shown in Table 2. For U-266, hybrids were produced in 38% of the seeded wells; however, only three secreted IgM. HMy$_2$ produced hybrids in 17% of the seeded wells and 67% of these hybrids secreted IgM. HF$_2$ produced hybrids in 46% of the seeded wells and 24% secreted IgM. UC729-6 yielded hybrids in 51% of the seeded wells, and 43% secreted IgM. Hybrids formed with the latter two cell lines were ready for testing on day 14, while hybrids from U-266 and HMy$_2$ were ready on days 32 and 20, respectively. Neither RPMI 8226 nor GM4672 yielded hybrid growth in these experiments. The murine NS-1 line produced hybrids in 80% of the seeded wells with 60% secreting IgM.

Results of cloning are also shown in Table 2. None of the originally positive wells from fusions with U-266 were cloned successfully; although clones did grow, none maintained secretion of IgM. All three wells from the HMy$_2$ fusions selected for cloning grew hybrid clones, but secretion was maintained in the clones from only one of these wells. Similarly, 1/9 originally positive wells from fusions with HF$_2$ and 2/8 from fusions with UC729-6 produced clones that maintained secretion of IgM. Two of six originally positive wells from fusions with the murine myeloma line NS-1 maintained secretion after cloning.

Comparison of immunoglobulin secretion by the cloned hybrids are shown in Table 3. The human-murine fusion

TABLE 2. Summary of Results of Three Separate Fusions of CLL Cells With Human Lines

Parent cell line

Fusion	U-266	HMy$_2$	HF$_2$	UC729-6	GM4672	RPMI 8226	NS-1
Wells seeded	968	880	1012	846	804	1012	352
Wells with growth in HAT	264	132	485	422	0	0	270
% Hybrids[a]	38	17	46	51	0	0	80
Secretors[b]	3	88	130	179	0	0	164
% Secretors among hybrids[c]	1	67	24	43	0	0	60
Hybrids cloned	3	3	9	8	0	0	6
Cloned hybrid secretors	0	1	1	2	0	0	1
% Stable clones[d]	0	33	11	25	0	0	17

[a]Number of hybrids/number of wells seeded X 100.
[b]Optical density $\geq$ 30% of positive control (100 ng/well of IgMk).
[c]Number of hybrids secreting IgM/number of hybrids X 100.
[d]Number of clones secreting IgM/number of hybrids cloned X 100.

secreted the highest level of human immunoglobulin, followed
by the UC729-6, HF_2 and HMy_2 hybrids, respectively. The
clones derived from the human-human fusions have continued to
secrete immunoglobulin for longer than twenty weeks, when
production of immunoglobulin by the human-mouse clone ceased.

TABLE 3.   Secretion of Antibody by Hybrid Clones

Clone	Parent Cell Line	Human IgM Antibody Secretion ($\mu g/ml/10^6$ cells)*
7D7G9	UC729-6	1.6
7D7A9	HF_2	1.3
7D7B3	HMy_2	0.8
80-13	NS-1	2.4

* Only the most productive clone was selected for analysis
when more than one were available.

B.   In Vitro Sensitization

When human lymphoid cells were cultured with 1ng/ml
tetanus toxoid in 1ml cultures, antibody could be detected by
the ELISA assay on day 6 or 7. Antibody production peaked at
day 11 or 12 and then declined. The maximum IgG production
peaked at 9.3ng/ml. Of the five donors tested, three produced
antibody exclusively of the IgG class, and two produced both
IgG and IgM, although the IgG titer was always much higher.
There was no apparent correlation between the time of the last
tetanus toxoid booster injection and the antibody class(es)
produced. In cultures lacking the antigen, no specific antibody was observed. Also, no antibody against noncross-
reacting antigens such as keyhole limpet hemocyanin and diphtheria toxoid could be measured.

C.   Hybridoma Production

The production of hybridomas which secrete human antibodies directed against tetanus toxoid was achieved by fusing
cells immunized in vitro for as little as six days (Table 4).

The efficiency of successful hybridoma formation increased from 1/24 positive wells using six day-sensitized cells to 8/24 positives using cells immunized for ten days. Thus, in vitro-sensitized cells were better fusion partners for hybridoma production just prior to the time of maximal antibody secretion.

TABLE 4.   Antibody Secretion of Human-Human Fusions From In Vitro Immunized Peripheral Blood Cultures

Days of Culture Prior to Fusion	Percent Positive Wells*	
	IgM	IgG
6	0 (0/24)	4 (1/24)
7	0 (0/24)	4 (1/24)
8	4 (1/24)	8 (2/24)
9	13 (3/24)	29 (7/24)
10	8 (2/24)	33 (8/24)

* Wells producing anti-tetanus toxoid antibody at day 28 post-fusion.

The relative amount of antibody secreted by the hybridoma cultures did not differ significantly with regard to the sensitization time of the lymphoid cells (Figure 1). Those cultures which showed IgM production always did so at very low, but measurable, levels. IgG production was much greater, although there was considerable variation in titer among the different culture wells of fused cells.

The hybrids produced were products of individual clones, as shown by repeated limiting dilution assay. The probability that any culture was propagated from multiple clones was less than 0.001 by Poisson statistical analysis.

The IgG-producing hybrids have tended to be relatively stable antibody producers. The cloned hybrids maintained antibody production for at least 120 days, with a relatively constant rate of antibody synthesis. At this point, however, antibody production ceased.

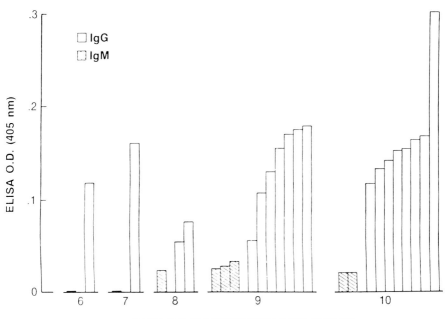

DAYS OF CULTURE PRIOR TO FUSION

FIGURE 1.   Antibody production of human hybridomas.   The
human blood cells (from a single individual) were immunized in
vitro against tetanus toxoid for 6-10 days prior to fusion
with U-266.   The successful fusions (c.f. Table 4) were tested
for level of specific antibody production by ELISA at day 28
following fusion.   An O.D. value of 0.2 units corresponds to
approximately 200ng specific antibody per ml.

IV. DISCUSSION

A. Comparison of Human Lines for Hybridoma Production

Although the rate of hybrid formation with U-266 was appreciable, only three hybrids secreted IgM. This was the same parental cell line employed by Olsson and Kaplan (2), although this mutant was independently derived. No hybrids were produced in 3/3 experiments with cell lines RPMI 8226 nor GM4672 (Table 2). RPMI 8226 has been previously used in our laboratory in ten fusions with non-CLL human cells, and hybrid formation occurred in 0 to 50%. Following in vitro sensitization of human lymphocytes with tetanus toxoid, we were able to achieve specific antibody secretion in 33% of the hybrids produced with U-266 (9) (results shown above). Croce et al. used lymphocytes from a patient with severe subacute sclerosing panencephalitis to produce anti-measles monoclonal antibodies with GM4672 (2). It is possible that these three cell lines require highly sensitized lymphocytes (the equivalent of the hyperimmunized mouse splenocyte) in order to form hybrids successfully. It is also possible that use of different fusion protocols would improve the fusion efficiency of these cells with the CLL cells used in this experiment.

Fusions with HMy_2 yielded hybrids in only 17% of the seeded wells, but 67% of the hybrids secreted immunoglobulin. Further investigations involving use of different fusion protocols and/or different molecular weight polyethylene glycols to increase hybrid efficiency would be justified with this line, because of this high percentage of hybrids producing immunoglobulin. Furthermore, successful fusions with this line have been reported (10). Fusions with UC729-6 and its clone, HF_2, produced hybrids in 51% and 46% of the seeded wells, with immunoglobulin secretion in 43% and 24%, respectively. It is likely that the fusion protocol employed to produce this substantial number of hybrids is sufficient and that further investigations with these lines should be devoted to a study of factors that might improve immunoglobulin secretion.

It is encouraging that human lines UC729-6 and HF_2 yielded results that were nearly equivalent to those obtained with NS-1, a well established murine myeloma cell line. The advantage of the human lines may be stability of secretion. It was, however, discouraging to find that the majority of the hybrids lost immunoglobulin secretion in the first stage of cloning (Table 2). Although the most likely reason for loss of this differentiated function in human-mouse fusions is rapid exclusion of human chromosomes, it is possible that loss

of immunoglobulin secretion in the human-human fusions is due
to an entirely different mechanism, such as a switching off of
gene function, or a loss of secretion, but not production.
Indeed, because the human CLL cell is not a normal B cell
secreting immunoglobulin in response to a known antigen, it is
possible that better equivalents to the hyperimmunized murine
splenocyte would carry genetic information capable of maintaining the function of antibody secretion after fusion.

B. Development of Human Hybridomas Using In Vitro-
    Sensitized Human Cells as Fusing Partners

The extension of in vitro sensitization to using these
in vitro-sensitized cells as fusion partners is relatively
straightforward. Success in such an endeavor, as reported
here, depends on the ability to reliably perform human sensi-
tizations, and to successfully fuse with a suitable human
myeloma or B lymphoblastoid line. The experiments described
above might suggest that we would have had even greater success using the HF_2 or the UC729-6 line.

In vitro sensitization not only gave us specific antibody
production from the hybridomas, it significantly increased the
number of successful fusion events. In our experience, about
3% to 10% of wells from fusions of hyperimmunized murine
spleen cells make the desired antibody, whereas we observed up
to 33% specific antibody-producing hybrids following in vitro
immunization. This may be due to selection events during
culture, favoring the expansion of the relevant B cell clones.
Also, the fusions reported here involved only about ten million lymphoid cells in each case, with an equal number of
myeloma parent cells. This is far fewer cells than the number
typically used in murine fusions, and makes feasible the use
of small amounts of human peripheral blood as the source of
the lymphocytes for fusion.

The in vitro system described here probably represents a
secondary immunization reponse, since the lymphocyte donors
all had been previously immunized with tetanus toxoid and some
had received recent booster inoculations. This may in part
account for the predominance of IgG antibody production, as
opposed to IgM production. This provides direct evidence that
memory cells committed to particular antigens remain in the
peripheral circulation for long periods of time, and that they
can be activated and clonally expanded in vitro.

We are currently using this in vitro procedure to enhance
the development of hybridomas producing antibodies to human
tumor-associated antigens. These methods should be generally
applicable to the production of human monoclonal antibodies to

a number of soluble and particulate antigens to obtain greater
yields of antigen-specific hybridomas using human peripheral
blood lymphoid cells as the source of cells for hybridoma
production. The success of this methodology paves the way for
the production of autologous monoclonal antibodies which may
react against tumor-associated antigens of cancer patients, as
these antigens are isolated and purified. This, in turn, will
offer a new modality for potential therapy with all the advantages of autologous material.

ACKNOWLEDGMENTS

We would like to thank Dr. R. Herberman for his advice and
counsel in critically reviewing this manuscript and S.
Pickeral and G. Clarke for technical assistance.

ABBREVIATIONS

CLL, chronic lymphocytic leukemia; ELISA, enzyme-linked
immunosorbent assay; EBV, Epstein-Barr virus.

REFERENCES

1. Croce, C.M., Linnenbach, A., Hall, W., Steplewski, Z.,
    and Koproski, H. Nature 288, 488 (1980).
2. Olsson, L. and Kaplan, H.S. Proc. Natl. Acad. Sci. USA
    77, 5429 (1980).
3. Köhler, G. and Milstein, C. Nature 256, 495 (1975).
4. Hatzubai, A., Maloney, D.G., and Levy, R. J. Immunol.
    126, 2397 (1981).
5. Miller, R.A., Maloney, D.G., Warnke, R., and Levy, R.
    New Eng. J. Med. 309, 517 (1982).
6. Lane, H.C., Volkman, D.J., Whalen, G., and Fauci, A.S.
    J. Exp. Med. 154, 1043 (1981).
7. Misiti, J. and Waldmann, T.A. J. Exp. Med. 154, 1069
    (1981).
8. Mishell, R.I. and Dutton, R.W. J. Exp. Med. 126, 423
    (1967).

9.   Rossio, J.L., Knost, J.A., Pickeral, S.F., and
     Abrams, P.D. J. Clin. Invest. (in press).
10. Sikora, K., Alderson, T., Phillips, J. and Watson, J.V.
     Lancet, January 2, 11 (1982).
11. Abrams, P.G., Knost, J.A., Clarke, G., Wilburn, S.,
     Oldham, R.K., and Foon, K.A. J. Immunol. (in press).

QUESTIONS AND ANSWERS

EDWARDS: Is your 8226 line human or rodent, because at least
two groups that have published fusions working with RPMI 8226
strains have subsequently found that their strain of RPMI 8226
was, in fact, a rodent line?

OLDHAM: Our line came from the American Type Culture Collection, but we have not karyotyped them in our lab.

EDWARDS: Both examples of 8226 that were rodent cells origin-
ated from the American Type Culture Collection.

OLDHAM: We will certainly check our cells when I get back.

HANDLEY: What was your method of producing the lymphokines
used in your in vitro immunization studies, and were your
dilutions those of supernatants?

OLDHAM: We used Con A-induced supernatants and diluted them
accordingly.

PRODUCTION OF STABLE HUMAN–HUMAN HYBRIDOMAS AT HIGH FREQUENCY[1]

Joy G. Heitzmann
Melvin Cohn

Developmental Biology Laboratory
The Salk Institute for Biological Studies
La Jolla, California

I. INTRODUCTION

We describe a new system for the rapid production at high frequency ($>10^{-5}$) of stable human hybridoma cells secreting high levels (5–30μg/ml) of human immunoglobulin. Mitogen-stimulated human B cells have been fused with WI-L2-729-HF$_2$, a high efficiency fusion variant of the thioguanine-resistant human lymphoblastoid cell line (1-3).[2] WI-L2-729-HF$_2$ cells produce trace levels of an IgG,κ (50–100ng/ml) and have surface IgM,κ. After fusion with tonsil or adenoid lymphocytes, stimulated in vitro by the B cell-specific mitogen, formalinized Staphylococcus aureus Cowan I strain (4,5), there is a rapid appearance (within two weeks) of hybridoma clones, all secreting new human immunoglobulin isotypes not detected in the parental WI-L2-729-HF$_2$ cell line, i.e. IgA or λ. These hybridoma clones have remained stable for five months (the longest period tested so far), producing high levels of new IgA and λ. As does the parental cell line, hybridoma cells grow and continue to secrete immunoglobulin in

---

[1]Supported by grants from the NIH (AI05875), the NMSS (RG1412-A-1), and the Kroc Foundation.
[2]WI-L2-729-HF$_2$ variant selected by Dr. R. Lundak at University of California, Riverside (present address: Techniclone, Santa Ana, CA).

serum-free medium[3], thereby facilitating possible large-scale production and purification of human antibodies. This system has the potential to provide tools and reagents for investigations involving, for example, the diagnosis and treatment of human autoimmune disease and cancer.

II. RESULTS AND DISCUSSION

WI-L2-729-HF$_2$ is a high efficiency fusion variant whose fusion frequency (10^{-5}-10^{-4}) is approximately 1000-fold greater than its parental cell line. WI-L2-729-HF$_2$ grows rapidly (about 18 hours doubling time) and dies quickly in selective hypoxanthine-aminopterin-thymidine (HAT) medium, allowing the rapid appearance and cloning of hybridomas (6). Normal human lymphocytes from nonimmunized donors were stimulated four days in vitro with .005-01% reformalinized (to prevent shedding soluble Protein A) Staphylococcus aureus Cowan I strain (4,5), a B cell-specific (T cell-independent) mitogen, to provide proliferating B cells. These were fused with WI-L2-729-HF$_2$ cells in 45% polyethylene glycol (PEG, MW 4000) containing 18% dimethyl sulfoxide (DMSO) in RPMI-1640 medium by standard procedures (7). Fused cells weie plated into either 2.0ml- or 0.2ml-well trays in HAT medium. Nonfused cells were plated separately or mixed as co-cultures into control wells. Preliminary experiments varied fusion parameters and conditions that influence fusion frequency and yield of stable hybridomas. Our present protocol stresses fusion in 45% PEG, 18% DMSO by incubation for six minutes at 37°C, fusion ratios (normal:tumor) of 2:1 or lower, and murine peritoneal macrophages as a feeder layer.

Typical fusions of WI-L2-729-HF$_2$ with tonsil or adenoid lymphocytes resulted in the rapid growth of HAT-resistant hybridomas within two weeks. Control wells were dead in HAT medium within one week. A plating density of approximately 2×10^6 fused cells per 2.0ml well yielded hybridomas in nearly every well, all of which were secreting new human Ig isotypes not synthesized by the WI-L2-729-HF$_2$ parental line (IgA or λ). Table 1 describes the human Ig chain analysis by enzyme-linked immunosorbent assay (ELISA) of hybridomas from 2.0ml wells of probable multiclonal origin. These results demonstrate high

---

[3]HB101 serum-free medium is available from Hana Media, Inc., a subsidiary of Hana Biologics, Inc., Berkeley, CA.

rates of secretion (89% secrete 5µg/ml or more). All wells were secreting new IgA and 86% were secreting new λ chain.

TABLE 1. ELISA Results of Macrowell Hybridomas*

Well Number	γ	µ	α	λ	κ
8	+	+	+	+	+
9	+	+	+	+	+
11	+	+	+	+	+
13	+	+	+	+	+
14	+	+	+	−	+
15	+	+	+	+	+
16	+	+	+	+	+
17	+	+	+	−	+
18	+	+	+	+	+
20	+	+	+	+	N.D.
21	+	+	+	+	+
22	+	+	+	+	N.D.
23	+	+	+	+	N.D.
25	+	+	+	+	+

*Supernatants from macrowell hybridomas were analyzed for human Ig by a modified ELISA (8,9). Briefly, 96-well plates (U-bottom polyvinyl) were sensitized with affinity-purified goat anti-human Ig (GaHIg polyvalent, GaHIgG, GaHIgM, GaHIgA, GaH λ Fab, or GaH κ Fab, obtained from Tago, Burlingame, CA). Specific binding by either hybridoma supernatants or HIg standards was detected by binding an alkaline phosphatase-GaHIg conjugate (Tago), whose reaction product with substrate was measured by optical density at 405nm (Artek automated plate reader). Quantities of <1ng are detected by this ELISA. WI-L2-729-HF$_2$ culture supernatants contain 50–100ng/ml IgG,κ; <50ng/ml IgM,κ; and no detectable IgA or λ. Positive wells (+) secrete specific Ig chains in µg/ml quantities. Negative wells (−) secrete no detectable Ig (i.e., λ chain). N.D. indicates ELISA results were not determined for some clones (i.e., κ chain).

The fusion frequency of the WI-L2-729-HF$_2$ hybridoma system was determined experimentally. Cells were fused at a 1:1 ratio and plated into seven microwell (0.2ml) trays at limiting dilution (5.0×10^5–5.0×10^4 cells per well). By day

15, wells were scored for growth of hybridoma clones. A significant decrease was observed when cells were plated at
$\langle 2.0 \times 10^5$ cells per well; above this plating density, 100% of
the wells were positive. These data demonstrate recovery of
one in 10^5-10^4 human lymphocytes as hybridomas when fused with
WI-L2-729-HF$_2$ cells.

In addition to providing determination of the fusion frequency $(\rangle 10^{-5})$, the limiting dilution experiment also provided
clones for human Ig analysis. Hybridomas from microwell trays
likely to be monoclonal in origin were analyzed by ELISA after
expansion into 2.0ml wells. Table 2 summarizes the results;

TABLE 2. ELISA Results of Microwell Hybridomas*

Clone	α	λ
4.1	+	+
4.2	+	−
4.3	+	−
4.4	+	+
4.5	+	−
4.6	+	+
4.9	+	−
4.10	+	+
4.11	+	−
4.12	+	+
4.13	+	−
4.14	+	+
4.15	−	+
5.2	+	+
5.3	+	+
5.4	−	+
5.7	+	+
5.8	+	+
6.2	−	+
6.3	+	+
6.4	−	+
6.5	+	−
6.6	+	+
7.3	+	+

*Random hybridoma clones from microwell trays (4-7) of
probable monoclonal origin were screened for human Ig secretion by ELISA. Negative clones (−) secrete no detectable Ig
(α or λ as indicated).

all clones (24/24) were secreting either new IgA or new λ; 20/24 were secreting new IgA; 17/24 were secreting new λ. These results demonstrate new antibody synthesis and secretion in all monoclonal hybridoma cultures tested.

WI-L2-729-HF$_2$ hybridomas have exhibited stable growth and secretion properties. A number of clones have been grown continuously in culture for five months (the longest period tested so far), continuing to secrete high levels of new Ig chains (10–20μg/ml). An additional advantage of the WI-L2-729-HF$_2$ system is that hybridomas grow in serum-free medium. WI-L2-729-HF$_2$ hybridomas continue to secrete high levels of immunoglobulin when grown in the absence of serum. We expect that this feature will facilitate the production and purification of large amounts of human antibodies for further investigations.

ABBREVIATIONS

HAT, hypoxanthine-aminopterin-thymidine; PEG, polyethylene glycol; DMSO, dimethyl sulfoxide; ELISA, enzyme-linked immunosorbent assay.

REFERENCES

1. Levy, J., Virolainen, M. and Defendi, V. Cancer 22, 517 (1968).
2. Levy, J., Buell, D., Creich, C., Hirshaut, Y. and Silverberg, H. J. Natl. Cancer Inst. 46, 647 (1971).
3. Lever, J., Nuki, G. and Seegmiller, J. Proc. Natl. Acad. Sci. USA 71, 2679 (1974).
4. Schuurman, R., Gelfand, E. and Dosch, H. J. Immunol. 125, 820 (1980).
5. Dosch, H., Schuurman, R. and Gelfand, E. J. Immunol. 125, 827 (1980).
6. Littlefield, J. Science 145, 709 (1964).
7. Fazekas de St. Groth, S. and Scheidegger, D. J. Immunol. Meth. 35, 1 (1980).
8. Engvail, E. and Perlmann, P. Immunochem. 8, 871 (1971).
9. Engvail, E. and Perlmann, P. J. Immunol. 109, 129 (1972).

QUESTIONS AND ANSWERS

KAPLAN: Is the lymphoblastoid WI-L2-729-HF$_2$ line positive for Epstein-Barr virus?

HEITZMANN: Although   WI-L2-729-HF$_2$ is   positive   for Epstein-Barr nuclear antigen, the cells do not produce virus. In our experiments, co-culture control wells never resulted in cell growth, thereby indicating unlikely transformation of lymphocytes by Epstein-Barr virus.   In addition, we are confident that purification of human antibodies, free of any possible contamination, will be possible using either ascites fluid or culture supernatants from hybridomas grown in serum-free medium.

REITHMÜELLER: Is the high incidence of IgA secreting hybridomas found with other sources of lymphocytes, e.g., peripheral blood?

HEITZMANN: The high incidence of IgA secreting hybridomas obtained may well reflect use of tonsil and adenoid tissue (very likely surgically removed because of recurrent bacterial infection).   We are in the midst of preparing and analyzing peripheral blood fusions, and cannot predict what the results will show.   Note that analysis of peripheral blood hybridomas will include assay for specific antibody activity, so that secretion of IgA will not be necessary as an indication of new Ig production, whereas fusions with tonsil and adenoid tissue involved nonimmunized donors.

HUMAN MONOCLONAL ANTIBODIES TO HUMAN CANCERS[1]

Mark C. Glassy, Harold H. Handley and Ivor Royston

Cancer Center, Department of Medicine
University of California, San Diego
La Jolla, California

D. Howard Lowe

Department of Surgery
University of California, San Diego
La Jolla, California

I. INTRODUCTION

Human monoclonal antibodies are likely to have advantages over murine monoclonal antibodies for therapeutic regimens. Recent clinical reports on the administration of murine monoclonal antibodies to cancer patients (1-3) have suggested some promise for the future use of monoclonal antibodies in human immunotherapy. However, murine monoclonal antibodies have been shown to induce human anti-mouse antibodies upon repeated injection into tumor-bearing patients (2,4), possibly reducing the efficacy of this therapy. Therefore, the production of the human monoclonal antibodies to tumor-associated antigens may prove more useful for tumor serotherapy.

The production of human monoclonal antibodies to human tumor-associated antigens would require the availability of human B lymphocytes sensitized to the host's own tumor. Recently, investigators have shown that B lymphocytes isolated from regional draining lymph nodes of cancer patients secrete antibodies which recognize the host's tumor (5,6). These B cells, immortalized through fusion, may serve as a constant

---

[1]This work was supported by University of California Cancer Research Coordinating Committee and Hybritech, Inc. grants.

source of antibody reactive with human tumor-associated anti-gens. Therefore, we fused lymphocytes from lymph nodes drain-ing tumors of the prostate, cervix and kidney with the murine myeloma cell line NS-1 or the human lymphoblastoid B cell line UC 729-6 (7) to generate human Ig-secreting hybridomas. Here, we describe three human monoclonal IgM antibodies which recog-nize determinants associated with cells of tumor origin.

II. MATERIALS AND METHODS

A. Fusion and Selection of Hybridomas

Lymph nodes, usually received within three hours after surgery, were teased with Nugent forceps in RPMI-1640 media and isolated lymphocytes were cultured overnight at 37°C in 5% CO_2 in RPMI-1640 with 10% fetal calf serum (FCS) and 2mM L-glutamine. Lymphocytes were counted and mixed at a ratio of 2:1 with either murine P3-NS-1-Ag4-1 or UC 729-6 (7), then fused with polyethylene glycol 1500 as described (7). All fused cells were plated at 1.0×10^5 cells/well without the use of feeder layers in Costar 96-well microtiter plates with hypoxanthine-aminopterin-thymidine (HAT)-supplemented (8) RPMI-1640 with 10% FCS and L-glutamine. Within 10-20 days, wells positive for hybridoma growth were assayed for human antibody production and their reactivity to a limited human cell panel by an enzyme immunoassay (EIA). Wells positive for reactivity were cloned by limiting dilution without the use of feeder layers and expanded for further study.

B. Enzyme Immunoassay

Human monoclonal antibodies and their reactivity to cells were detected by an EIA previously described (9). Briefly, 50µl of either a class-specific affinity-purified goat anti-human Ig (Tago, Burlingame, CA) or a 4×10^6 target cell/ml suspension was immobilized in triplicate wells of an immuno-filtration manifold. After washing three times with 0.3% gelatin in phosphate-buffered saline, 50µl of hybridoma super-natant were incubated thirty minutes at room temperature. Filters were then washed and incubated with 50µl of a class-specific horseradish peroxidase-conjugated goat anti-human Ig (Tago) for an additional thirty minutes. Filters were washed again and incubated with 150µl of a 400µg/ml solution of ortho-phenylenediamine in citrate buffer. 100µl from each well were then transferred to a new plate containing 50μl of 2.5 M H_2SO_4 and read on a Dynatek (Alexandria, VA) MR 580 micro-ELISA reader at 490nm.

C. Surface and Cytoplasmic Ig

Cell surface and cytoplasmic Ig were detected by indirect immunofluorescence microscopy using techniques and reagents previously described (10).

D. Relative DNA Content

Cells (1.0×10^6) were fixed in 70% ethanol for two hours, washed (500xg for ten minutes) and resuspended in 100μl of phosphate-buffered saline. One ml of 0.05mg/ml solution of propidium iodine (Sigma) was added to the cell suspension, incubated for fifteen minutes at 4°C and filtered through a 50 micron pore nylon mesh. Samples were analyzed on an Ortho-Cytofluorograf 50H equipped with a 488mm argon ion laser, 400mW.

III. RESULTS

Table 1 outlines the results of each fusion attempting to produce human monoclonal antibodies to tumor-associated antigens. The fusion yielding MGH7, a mouse-human hybridoma secreting a human monoclonal IgM reactive with prostate carcinoma cell lines, generated 61 growth-positive wells of 188 wells plated. Of these, 57.4% were positive for human Ig. It should be noted that some wells secreted more than one isotype. MGH7 was subcloned twice by limiting dilution when its human IgM was found to react with Ln-Cap, a human prostate carcinoma cell line.

The fusion producing CLNH5, a human-human hybridoma secreting a monoclonal IgMκ reactive with cervical carcinoma cell lines, generated six growth-positive wells of 80 wells plated. CLNH5 was cloned by limiting dilution when it was found to react with the Hela and CaSki cervical carcinoma cell lines.

WLNA6, a human-human hybridoma secreting a monoclonal IgM reactive with a carcinoma of the lung, resulted from a fusion producing 23 growth-positive wells out of 49 wells.

Table 2 lists some of the cellular characteristics of

TABLE 1.   Generation and Identification of Human Monoclonal Antibodies

Lymph Node Draining	Number of Lymphocytes Fused	Number of Wells Plated	Number of Wells Positive for Hybridomas	Hybrids Secreting Ig			Known Reactivity
				IgG	IgM	IgA	
Prostate Carcinoma	1.5x10⁷	188	61	9	29	1	1 (MHG7)
Cervical Carcinoma	7.7x10⁶	80	6	1	2	0	1 (CLNH5)
Wilm's Tumor	1.0x10⁷	49	23	1	22	0	1 (WLNA6)

UC 729-6 and selected human Ig-secreting hybridomas, MHG7,
CLNH5, and WLNA6. All hybridomas have continued to secrete
$3-5\mu g/ml$ of human Ig/10^6 cells for over nine months in continuous culture and doubled every 20-30 hours. The properties
of these hybridomas have remained unchanged after preservation
in liquid nitrogen and reconstitute reliably.

Cytofluorograf analysis of CLNH5 (Figure 1) showed this
hybridoma to be a pseudotetraploid human-human hybridoma and
not an Epstein-Barr virus (EBV)-transformed normal pseudo-
diploid lymphocyte transfected with EBV from UC 729-6. MHG7
appears to be a population of mouse-human hybrids that have
undergone a partial segregation of human chromosomes (11) and,
therefore, have a varying DNA content.

Table 3 lists the relative amounts of human monoclonal
antibody bound to each of the cell lines listed, as measured
by EIA. MHG7 reacted with carcinomas of prostate (Ln-Cap) and
lung origin (T293H) and was negative with carcinomas of the
cervix and lung, T leukemia, normal fibroblasts, and peripheral blood lymphocytes (PBL). CLNH5 showed positive reactivity with carcinomas of the cervix (CaSki, Hela), lung
(T293H, Calu-1, and SK-MES-1), fibroblasts, T leukemia, and
PBL (7). WLNA6 showed strong positive reactivity with lung
(T293H), weak reactivity with cervix (CaSki, Hela), and was

TABLE 2.   Cellular Characteristics of Human Ig-Secreting
           Hybridomas

Characteristics	UC 729-6	MHG 7	CLNH5	WLNA6
sIg	IgM$_\kappa$	IgM$_\kappa$	IgD, IgM$_\kappa$	NT
cyIg	IgM$_\kappa$	IgM	IgM	IgM
Chromosome Content	Diploid	Pseudo-tetraploid	Pseudo-tetraploid	Pseudo-tetraploid
Supernatant*				
IgA	<.05 µg	<.05 µg	<.05 µg	<.05 µg
IgG	<.05 µg	<.05 µg	<.05 µg	<.05 µg
IgM	<.05 µg	5.00 µg	5.00 µg	3.00 µg

* = Amount of Ig secreted/10^6 cells
NT = Not tested

negative for prostate (Ln-Cap), normal fibroblasts, and T leukemia.   All other human monoclonal antibodies generated were negative for the cell lines shown.

The results of indirect immunofluorescent staining for detection of the binding of MHG7 to several cases of prostate carcinoma and benign prostatic hypertrophy (BPH) are summarized in Table 4.   Both frozen sections and paraffin-embedded formalin sections gave positive results.   Eleven of seventeen cases of prostate carcinoma were positive for MHG7 in at least 5% of the tumor cell population.   Six of nine cases of BPH were MHG7 positive.   MHG7 did not react with normal prostate cells on both frozen and paraffin-embedded tissue sections.

IV. DISCUSSION

In this paper we describe the generation and identification of three human monoclonal antibodies recognizing antigenic determinants associated with tumor cells.   Since it has

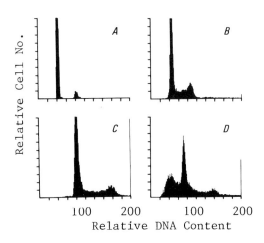

FIGURE 1.   Relative DNA Content of Chronic Lymphocytic
Leukemia (A), UC 729-6 (B), CLNH5.5 (C), and MHG7.M1 (D).
Cell number is plotted on the ordinate against relative fluo-
rescent intensity on the abscissa.

been suggested that humans make antibodies to their own tumors
(see reference 12 for a recent review), we fused lymphocytes
isolated from human lymph nodes which drain tumors (5,6) with
either NS-1 or UC 729-6 to immortalize these human antibody-
producing cells.   The three human monoclonal antibodies described here have, so far, preferentially reacted with cell
lines of tumor origin and not with normal fibroblasts, lymphoblastoid cell lines, or normal peripheral blood lymphocytes.
Of note, the MHG7 monoclonal antibody, derived from a lymph
node draining a prostate cancer, preferentially bound to
Ln-Cap, a prostate carcinoma cell line.   In addition, the
CLNH5 monoclonal antibody, derived from a lymph node draining
a cervical carcinoma, reacted with cervical carcinoma cell
lines.   Since these human monoclonal antibodies reacted with
some, but not all, of the tumor cell lines tested, more work
will be necessary before we can draw conclusions regarding the
utility of these monoclonal antibodies in discriminating tumor
cells from normal cell types.
     We have also demonstrated that the MHG7 monoclonal anti-
body bound to prostate carcinoma cells and hypertrophied prostate, but not normal prostate cells, on frozen and formalin-
fixed, paraffin-embedded tissue sections.   This data suggests

TABLE 3. Reactivity of Human Monoclonal Antibodies With Human Cell Lines

Cell Line	Type	$O.D_{490}$ Readings*		
		MGH7	CLNH5	WLNA6
CaLu-1	Lung Carcinoma	0.018	0.342	0.029
SK-MES-1	Lung Carcinoma	0.022	0.395	NT
T293H	Lung Carcinoma	0.132	0.498	0.753
Hela	Cervical Carcinoma	0.016	0.443	0.140
CaSki	Cervical Carcinoma	NT	0.429	0.145
Ln-Cap	Prostate Carcinoma	0.265	0.386	0.005
350Q	Normal Fibroblast	0.030	0.026	0.041
WI-38	Normal Fibroblast	0.026	0.038	0.033
CEM	T Leukemia	0.022	0.019	0.029

*$O.D_{490}$ readings were obtained utilizing a Dynatech micro-ELISA reader (model MR 580) in a quantitative immunofiltration assay (9). $O.D_{490}$ readings for each cell line with an irrelevant human monoclonal IgM were subtracted from the test results. NT = not done.

TABLE 4. Immunofluorescent Staining of Tissue Sections With MHG7

Tissue	# Cases Positive/ # Cases Tested		% Tumor Ducts Involved
	MHG7	Irrelevant IgM	
Frozen Sections			
Prostate Carcinoma	4/5	0/5	10-30%
Benign Prostatic Hypertrophy	2/3	0/3	25-35%
Normal Prostate	0/2	0/2	0%
Formalin-Fixed Sections			
Prostate Carcinoma	7/12	0/12	5-30%
Benign Prostatic Hypertrophy	4/6	0/6	5-30%
Foreskin	0/3	0/3	0%

that the antigen detected by MHG7 may represent a tumor-associated antigen. However, since BPH cells also reacted with MHG7, further work will be necessary to correlate antigen expression with the malignant state.

The production of human antibodies to tumor-associated antigens confirms the presence of lymphocytes in lymph nodes capable of producing tumor-reactive antibodies. Such human monoclonal antibodies may be useful in cancer immunotherapy pending further study of normal tissue reactivity.

ABBREVIATIONS

FCS, fetal calf serum; HAT, hypoxanthine-aminopterin-thymidine; EIA, enzyme immunoassay; EBV, Epstein-Barr virus; BPH, benign prostatic hypertrophy.

REFERENCES

1. Dillman, R.O., Shawler, D.L., Sobol, R.E., Collins, H.A., Beauregard, J.C., Wormsley, W.B. and Royston, I.   Blood 39, 1036 (1982).
2. Miller, R.A., Maloney, D.G., Warnke, R. and Levy, R.   New Engl. J. Med. 306, 517 (1982).
3. Ritz, J., Pesanda, J.M., Sallan, SE., Clavell, L.A., Notis-McOnarty, J., Rosenthal, P. and Schlossman, S.F. Blood 58, 151 (1981).
4. Dillman, R.O., Shawler, D.L., Beauregard, J.C., Wormsley, S.B. and Royston, I.   Blood 60, 161a (1982).
5. Schlom, J., Wunderlich, D., Teramoto, R.A.   Proc. Natl. Acad. Sci. USA 77, 6841 (1980).
6. Sikora, K. and Wright, R.   Br. J. Cancer 43, 696 (1981).
7. Handley, H.H. and Royston, I., in 'Hybridomas in Cancer Diagnosis and Treatment' (M. Mitchell and H. Oettgen, eds.), p. 124, Raven Press, New York (1982).
8. Littlefield, J.W.   Science 145, 709 (1964).
9. Glassy, M.C., Handley, H.H., Cleveland, P.H. and Royston, I.   J. Immunol. Meth. 58, 119 (1983).
10. Royston, I., Majda, J.A., Baird, SM., Meserve, B.L., and Griffiths, J.C.   J. Immunol. 125, 715 (1980).
11. Ruddle, R.   Nature 242, 165 (1973).
12. Hellstrom, K.E., Brown, J.P., in 'The Antigens', Vol. V (M. Sela, ed.), p. 1-96, Academic Press, New York (1979).

THE CLINICAL POTENTIAL OF HUMAN
MONOCLONAL ANTIBODIES IN ONCOLOGY

Karol Sikora, Thomas Alderson and Howard Smedley

Ludwig Institute for Cancer Research
MRC Centre, Hills Road
Cambridge, United Kingdom

I. INTRODUCTION

Monoclonal antibodies allow the precise definition of individual components of complex antigenic structures, such as tumor cell surfaces. Mouse and rat monoclonal antibodies raised against human tumor cells have identified molecules that are present in greater quantity on tumors when compared with normal cells (1). Such antibodies have already been shown to have clinical use in diagnosis by providing markers of tumor load and for radiolocalization of tumor deposits. Promising preliminary results in therapeutic trials with these antibodies in patients with colorectal cancer (2) and nodular lymphoma (3) have recently been reported. A major problem with such antibodies has been their lack of specificity. Although the target antigens recognized may often be expressed in increased quantities on tumor cells, most monoclonal antibodies show no absolute tumor specificity. Many of the antigens are present in small quantities on stem cells in normal tissue. The xenogeneic immunization schedules used in the preparation of these monoclonal antibodies emphasize certain components on the cell surface, such as the blood group substances and histocompatibility antigens, which are shared by normal and neoplastic cells. A further problem with xenogeneic monoclonal antibodies is the immune response to them when used clinically, which may abrogate their effects. Furthermore, they tell us nothing about the way in which the

171

host's immune system is responding to the presence of autologous tumor.

There is considerable evidence that patients are able to
mount a serological response to their own neoplastic cells, at
least in some stages in the natural history of their disease
(4). By fusing lymphocytes likely to be involved in this
response with a suitable myeloma line, hybridomas can be produced and antibody activity analyzed. Several human systems
have now been described in the literature. We have chosen to
use the LON-LICR HMy2 line (5) in our attempts to make human
monoclonal antibodies to a wide range of tumor types using
lymphocytes from several sources. Peripheral blood, regional
lymph node, and intratumoral lymphocytes have been collected
and fused. After cloning, the supernatants were screened for
antitumor activity on cell lines. Twelve antibodies were
obtained which bound significantly to tumor cells but not to
normal fibroblasts, lymphocytes or red cells. Two of these
were labeled with ^{131}I and used in attempts to localize tumors
in patients.

To study the feasibility of continuous administration of
human monoclonal antibodies directed against glioma we
designed a chamber which enables hybridoma cells to be cultured in the subcutaneous tissue (6). This chamber allows
antibodies to diffuse out and nutrients and oxygen necessary
for continued cell viability to diffuse in. Cells are unable
to traverse the membrane pores of the device, so there is no
risk that malignant cells put in the chamber can metastasize.
The chamber has now been inserted into one patient with recurrent glioma, in whom the kinetics of internally labeled antibody release have been monitored.

II. METHODS

A. Monoclonal Antibody Preparation and Assay

We collected tumor material and regional lymph nodes from
patients having surgery for a variety of tumor types. Cell
fusion was carried out using polyethylene glycol (PEG) (7).
Following dilution cloning, the immunoglobulins secreted by
the hybridomas were assayed using a sensitive radioimmunassay
using Ig chain-specific mouse monoclonal antibodies (8). DNA
content of the hybridomas was determined using a flow cyto-
meter (9). A variety of human tumor cell lines were used to
assess binding activity in an indirect radioimmunoassay.

B. Tumor Localization

Hybridomas were grown in Iscove's medium, and the supernatant precipitated in $(NH_4)_2SO_4$ (50%). The washed
precipitate was dissolved in phosphate-buffered saline and the
Ig purified using a protein A-Sepharose column. Purified Ig
was labeled with ^{131}I (1mCi/mg) by a modified chloramine-T
method. 1mg of labeled monoclonal antibody was administered
i.v. in 20ml normal saline to one patient with recurrent
glioma and three patients with bronchial carcinoma.

C. The Chamber

A cylindrical diffusion chamber was constructed of
'Delrin', a synthetic homopolymer. The upper section contained an outlet and inlet hole into which were inserted 21-
gauge needles. This assembly screws into the lower cylindrical section which has an internal and external flange at the
base. The internal flange holds a 3cm diameter injection-
molded 'Millipore' filter. The external flange enables the
chamber to be immobilized in the subcutaneous tissue. The
filter allows the free diffusion of large molecules, but not
of cells, between the chamber and the patient's extracellular
fluid (Figure 1).

III. RESULTS

A. Cell Fusion

Clinical material was obtained from 180 patients with a
variety of tumor types (Table 1). Apparently successful initial fusion was observed in 55 patients. Low lymphocyte
yields and infection were the major problems in the initial
stages. Once established, hybridomas were rapidly growing
with doubling times of 24-36 hours. All hybrids tested were
easily adapted for growth in serum-free (Iscove's) medium in
4-liter roller bottles. Evidence of hybridization was
obtained by detecting an increase in DNA content on flow cytometry and morphological changes on electron microscopy.

B. Immunoglobulin Secretion

All hybridomas continued to produce the kappa and gamma
chains secreted by HMy2. In addition, 14% produced λ chains,

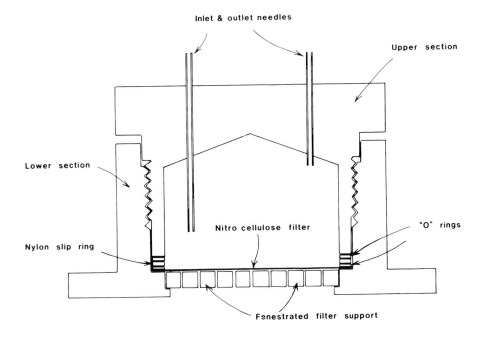

FIGURE 1. The Diffusion Chamber.

15% μ chains, 13% α chains and 1% ε chains. The production of new immunoglobulins continued after prolonged tissue culture. 1-5μg/ml of immunoglobulin were detected in the supernatants.

C. Antitumor Antibody Activity and Specificity

Antibodies were initially screened for binding activity against the cell line most appropriate to the source of donor lymphocyte. Despite the sensitivity of the binding assay, the counts bound were low. After concentration, however, titration curves were obtained. These curves show only weak binding of antibody. However, the binding was significantly above

TABLE 1. Human Hybridoma Production

Tumor	Samples Processed	Lymphocyte Origin*	Successful Fusion	Patients With Hybrids	Total Hybrids
Lung	14	RN	8	2	27
Breast	29	RN	13	4	28
Colorectal	42	RN	12	3	6
Glioma	39	IT	18	9	84
Kidney	3	RN	0	0	0
Sarcoma	2	IT	0	0	0
Melanoma	2	RN	1	1	1
Uterus	13	RN	5	2	7
Stomach	14	RN	5	1	7
Bladder	18	RN	0	0	0
Burkitts	4	PB	3	2	2

* RN = regional node; IT = intratumoral; PB = peripheral blood

background when compared to that of HMy2 immunoglobulin at similar concentration. The specificity of binding was determined using several tumor cell lines (Table 2). Peripheral blood lymphocytes and red blood cells from normal donors were used as controls. It can be seen that all the antibodies isolated so far bind to a variety of cell types and are not specific for an individual tumor. A more precise definition of specificity was attempted using immunohistological methods on fresh frozen biopsies of tumor and normal tissue. No significant binding above background was observed. Indirect immunofluorescence on cell lines demonstrated similar binding specificity as seen in radioimmunoassay.

TABLE 2. Binding of Monoclonal Antibodies to Tumor Cell Lines

Supernatant	G/CCM	HT 29	MOR	CALU1	MCF7	MRC5	PBL	RBC
Glioma								
LGL1-1C3	+++	++	+	−	+++	−	−	−
LGL1-1C6	+++	++	+	−	++	−	±	−
LGL1-1D6	++	+	++	+	+	−	−	±
LGL1-2C1	++	++	+	+	−	±	−	±
LGL7-1A2	++	+	+	−	+	±	−	±
LGL7-3A2	++	+	+	++	−	−	−	−
LGL10-3B5	++	+	+	−	++	−	−	−
LGL22-4D6	++	+	++	+	+	−	−	±
Lung								
LLU1-3D1	++	++	++	++	+	−	−	−
LLU6-1A1	++	+	++	++	+	±	−	±
LLU6-2A4	++	+	+	+	−	−	−	−
LLU6-3D4	++	+	++	++	+	−	−	−

PBL = peripheral blood lymphocytes
RBC = red blood cells

D. Tumor Localization

1. Glioma

Figure 2 shows the radioactivity in serum, CSF and tumor cyst fluid following the i.v. administration of LGL1-1D6 and control IgG to a patient with recurrent glioma. There was no

FIGURE 2a and 2b. Radioactivity in serum, CSF and Tumor Cyst Fluid Following Intravenous Administration of LGL1-1DG and Control IgG. ●, serum; Δ, tumor cyst fluid; o, CSF; MCA = monoclonal antibody.

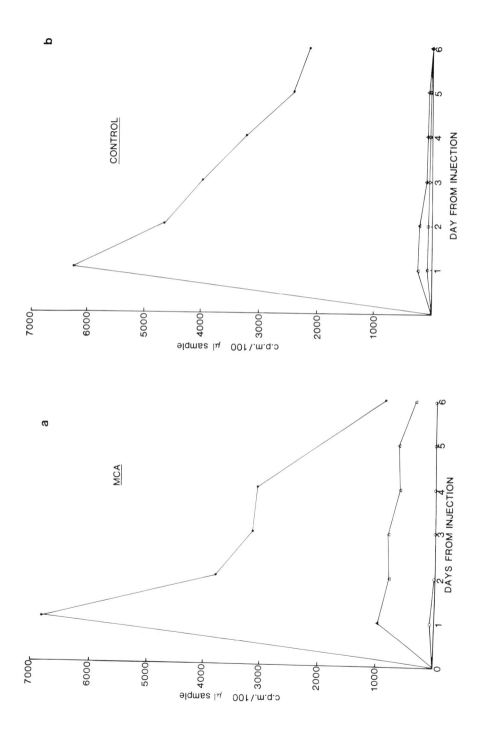

significant difference between counts in the serum or CSF
after the administration of labeled monoclonal antibody or
control IgG. However, the ^{131}I-labeled monoclonal antibody
persisted within the tumor cyst fluid for over six days. External counting over the cranial cavity and heart was performed. Tumor localization clearly occurred using the labeled
monoclonal antibody (Figure 3). Although disturbances in the
blood-brain barrier around an infiltrating tumor may result in
increased access to the tumor fluid by a range of serum
proteins, we demonstrated considerable differences between the
behavior of monoclonal antibody and control IgG.

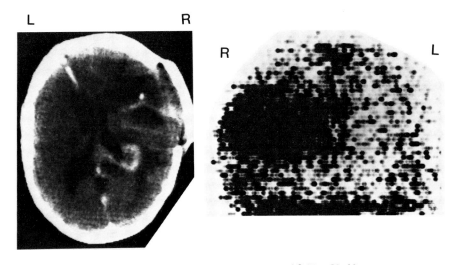

CT   SCAN   131I   McAb

FIGURE 3. Tumor Localization by McAb in a Patient With
Recurrent Glioma. McAb = monoclonal antibody.

2. Lung Cancer.

LLU6-2A4 was similarly labeled with ^{131}I and 1mg was given
i.v. to three patients with bronchial carcinoma. Using a
subtraction technique to remove the blood pool image (10),
scans were obtained which demonstrated the distribution of
tumor in two out of three patients.

E. Long-Term Administration

10^7 hybridoma cells which were pulse-labeled with 100μCi L-$(4,5-^3H)$ lysine monohydrochloride (specific activity 80Ci/mmol) were also placed in the chamber. Serum samples were collected from the patient at regular intervals after the insertion of the chamber, and trichloroacetic acid-precipitable ^3H counts were determined by scintillation counting. Release of tritiated monoclonal antibody from the chamber into the blood stream occurred in the three days after injection of pulse-labeled cells into the chamber. Intact, labeled antibody was detected in the tumor cyst fluid. The device remained in situ for three months and caused no problems – there has been no evidence of infection or of an inflammatory response around the chamber and no evidence of spread of hybridoma cells outside the chamber. There was no change in the patient's serum Epstein-Barr titer. We believe that this device can be used to study the long-term effects of this and other monoclonal antibodies.

IV. DISCUSSION

We have demonstrated that lymphocytes from patients with several tumor types can be successfully fused with a human lymphoid line to produce stable hybridomas. These hybridomas secrete immunoglobulins, several of which have been found to show weak binding to tumor cell lines in an indirect radioimmunoassay. Evidence for hybridization, rather than outgrowth of lymphoblastoid lines from the lymphocytes of patients, is provided by the continued secretion of HMy2 Ig as well as the new lymphocyte Ig in cloned hybridomas. Flow cytometric DNA analysis shows an increase in DNA content characteristic of hybrids. Formal karyotypic analysis has been performed on hybridomas derived from HMy2 which confirms an increase in chromosome number. The specificity studies on twelve antibodies clearly show a wide range of weak binding to different tumor cell lines. It is of interest that none of the antibodies bound to the benign fibroblast line (MRC-5), normal red cells, or peripheral blood lymphocytes. Our attempts to localize the antigens by immunohistological techniques in tissue sections have so far been unsuccessful due to a combination of weak binding and high background immunoglobulin in human tissues. We are beginning to use these antibodies for the clinical localization of tumors in patients with glioma and lung cancer.

ABBREVIATIONS

PEG, polyethylene glycol.

REFERENCES

1. Lennox, E.S. and Sikora, K. In 'Monoclonal Antibodies in Clinical Medicine' (A. McMichael and J. Fabre, eds.), p. 111. Academic Press, London (1982).

2. Sears, H.F., Atkinson, B., Mattis, J., Ernst, L., Herlyn, D., Steplewski, Z., Hayry, P. and Koprowski, H. Lancet, April 3, 762 (1982).

3. Miller, R.A., Maloney, D.G., Warnke, R. and Levy, R. New Eng. J. Med. 306, 517 (1982).

4. Shiku, H., Takahasti, T., Rednick, L., Oettgen, H. and Old, L.J. J. Exp. Med. 145, 784 (1977).

5. Edwards, P.A.W., Smith, C.M., Neville, A. and O'Hare, M.J. Eur. J. Immunol. 45, 61 (1982).

6. Watson, J.V., Alderson, T., Sikora, K. and Phillips, J. Lancet, January 15, 99 (1983).

7. Sikora, K., Alderson, T., Ellis, J., Phillips, J. and Watson, J. Br. J. Cancer 47, 135 (1983).

8. Sikora, K., Alderson, T. and Ellis, J. J. Immunol. Meth. 57, 151 (1983).

9. Watson, J.V. Cytometry, 1, 14 (1981).

10. Smedley, H., Finan, P., Lennox, E., Sikora, K. and Wraight, E. Br. J. Cancer 47, 253 (1983).

HUMAN-HUMAN HYBRIDOMAS

Paul A. W. Edwards,
Michael J. O'Hare and A. Munro Neville

Ludwig Institute for Cancer Research (London Branch)
Royal Marsden Hospital
Sutton, Surrey, United Kingdom

I. INTRODUCTION

Do human monoclonal antibodies, as compared to rodent monoclonal antibodies, have a role to play in the diagnosis and therapy of cancer? It is generally considered that human monoclonal antibodies will be needed for therapy to avoid an immune response to the injected antibody by the patient. However, it may be that patients could be rendered immunologically tolerant to mouse immunoglobulin; and, in any case, if an antibody is conjugated to a toxin, for example, this will presumably be immunogenic regardless of the species of immunoglobulin used. It is possible that the antigens recognized by the human immune system may be different from those most frequently recognized by antibodies raised in mouse hybridizations, but this remains to be demonstrated. In the meanwhile, the first priority is to establish a routine method that will generate large numbers of human monoclonal antibodies.

Human-human hybridoma systems have aroused much skepticism and controversy, not without justification. The original SKO-007 line (1) was infected with mycoplasma, though this has been cured (2,3). Fusions performed with Epstein-Barr nuclear antigen-positive lymphoblastoid lines (4-6) had to be shown convincingly to produce genuine hybrids rather than Epstein-Barr virus transformants. Cell lines purporting to be derived from the human myeloma line RPMI 8226 have been hybridized (7,8), but it is thought that both lines have nonhuman karyotype (9).

181

II. RESULTS

We have established and extensively characterized (5,10) a human-human hybridoma system based on the line LICR-LON-HMy2, which we derived from the lymphoblastoid line ARH-77 (12; see also 5). The line can be reproducibly hybridized with human lymphocytes. The cell lines obtained have been shown to be true hybrids (5,10) by secretion of immunoglobulin chains from both the lymphocyte hybridized and HMy2 after cloning, by karyotype and DNA content, and by HLA typing. Particular virtues of the HMy2 line are its robustness in culture (it grows rapidly, clones and freezes easily and is very tolerant of overgrowth or overdilution in culture) and its ability to hybridize reproducibly in several independent laboratories (11 and R. Cote and A. Houghton, cited in 3). Its limitations as presently seen include a low yield of hybrids compared to mouse hybridizations, though other laboratories report that it compares well with other human systems. In addition, it produces IgG1 with a kappa light chain so that hybrids produce these parental immunoglobulin chains, and many of the hybrids produce only 1 or 2µg/ml immunoglobulin in the medium at routine subculture, though a few cloned hybrids produce 4 to 16µg/ml. We are currently using it to hybridize with lymphocytes from lymph nodes draining breast tumors.

III. CONCLUSIONS

With the current state of the art, making human monoclonal antibodies is clearly more difficult than making mouse monoclonal antibodies, and even when fusion (or Epstein-Barr virus transformation) techniques improve, there will still be the problem of obtaining and selecting lymphocytes that have been immunized to antigens of interest. In the long run, the best method will probably be through in vitro immunization using a defined antigen. Recently some progress has been made in obtaining human responses in vitro (13), and recent advances in propagating T helper cell clones, construction of T cell hybridomas and understanding of T cell growth factors should provide considerable impetus to the development of practical methods.

At present, therefore, we believe that the most productive strategy is to concentrate on developing antibody-directed therapy with mouse monoclonal antibodies, using them to study such problems as the correct way to deal with antigenic heterogeneity and antigenic modulation, and to develop methods to assess destruction of tumor cells in vivo. When an ideal target antigen for antibody therapy has been identified, in vitro immunization could be used for controlled human hybridoma generation.

ACKNOWLEDGMENTS

We thank Isobel Brooks, Elizabeth Dinsdale and Clare Smith for excellent assistance.

REFERENCES

1. Olsson, L. and Kaplan, H.S.   Proc. Natl. Acad. Sci. USA 77, 5429 (1980).
2. Kaplan, H.S., Olsson, L., Reese, J. and Bieber, M. Hybridoma 1, 178 (1982).
3. Sikora, K. and Neville, A.M.   Nature (News and Views) 300, 316 (1982).
4. Croce, C.M., Linnenbach, A., Hall, W., Steplewski, Z. and Koprowski, H.   Nature 288, 488 (1980).
5. Edwards, P.A.W., Smith, C.M., Neville, A.M. and O'Hare, M.J.   Eur. J. Immunol. 12, 641 (1982).
6. Handley, H.H. and Royston, I.   In 'Hybridomas in Cancer Diagnosis and Treatment' (M.S. Mitchell and H.F. Oettgen, eds.), p. 125.   Raven Press, New York (1982).
7. Clark, S.A., Stimson, W..H., Williamson, A.R. and Dick, H.M.   J. Supramol. Struct. Cell. Biochem. Suppl. 5, 100a (1981).
8. Pickering, J.W. and Gelder, F.B.   J. Immunol. 129, 406 (1982).
9. Pickering, J.W. and Gelder, F.B.   J. Immunol. 129, 2314 (1982).
10. O'Hare, M.J., Smith, C.M. and Edwards, P.A.W.   In 'Protides of the Biological Fluids, Colloquium 30' (H. Peeters, ed.), p. 265.   Pergamon Press, Oxford (1983).

11. Sikora, K., Alderson, T., Phillips, J. and Watson, J.V. Lancet, January 2, 11 (1982).
12. Burk, K.J., Drewinko, B., Trujillo, J.M. and Ahearn, M.J. Cancer Res. 38, 2508 (1978).
13. Lane, H.C., Volkman, D.J., Whalen, G. and Fauci, A.S. J. Exp. Med. 154, 1043 (1981).

DIAGNOSIS II

IMMUNOHISTOLOGICAL ANALYSIS OF HUMAN MALIGNANCIES WITH MONOCLONAL ANTIBODIES[1]

David Y. Mason and Kevin C. Gatter

Nuffield Department of Pathology
University of Oxford, United Kingdom

I. INTRODUCTION

Immunohistological studies of human malignancies performed in the past, prior to the advent of monoclonal antibodies, were hampered by two major practical restrictions: (1) the high level of background staining and the frequency of nonspecific reactions associated with the use of polyclonal antisera, and (2) the restricted range of antigenic tissue constituents which could be detected with available antisera. Monoclonal antibodies have gone a long way towards removing both of these obstacles, and in the past two years the authors have used them extensively for the immunohistological analysis of lymphoid and epithelial neoplasms. In the present paper some of the points which have emerged from this work are briefly described.

II. MATERIALS AND METHODS

A. Tissue Section Preparation

The majority of these studies have been performed using cryostat sections (5μ in thickness) prepared from snap–frozen, unfixed tissue. Sections are thoroughly dried, fixed for ten

---

[1]Supported by grants from the Leukaemia Research Fund, the Wellcome Trust and the Cancer Research Campaign.

minutes in acetone at room temperature and then stored (if not
stained immediately) at -20°C.

B. Staining Procedure

In the authors' experience, most monoclonal antibodies
give satisfactory immunohistological labeling of tissue sections when used in a two-stage indirect immunoperoxidase procedure. The monoclonal antibody is applied for 30-60 minutes
and followed (after washing) by peroxidase-conjugated rabbit
anti-mouse Ig (Dako). This reagent is diluted 1/50 in Tris-
buffered saline (pH 7.6) containing 5% normal human serum (to
block cross-reactivity against human Ig). After thirty minutes incubation, sections are washed and the sites of antibody
binding revealed in a conventional manner using diaminobenzi-
dine and H_2O_2 as substrate. Only occasionally has it been
found necessary to increase the sensitivity of labeling, e.g.,
by using a three-stage immunoperoxidase procedure.

III. RESULTS AND DISCUSSION

A. Heterogeneity of Antigen Expression

A striking characteristic of many of the antigens detected
in human epithelial neoplasms is that their expression often
shows marked variation in intensity between different areas of
the tumor. An example of one antigen which commonly shows
this phenomenon (transferrin receptor) is illustrated in
Figure 1. However, other antigens also frequently show
heterogeneous patterns of expression on epithelial tumors,
including HLA Class 1 and 2 antigens, keratin-associated

FIGURE 1. (a): Immunoperoxidase labeling of a human
cutaneous basal cell carcinoma for transferrin receptor. The
neoplasm is strongly stained for this constituent, but negative lacunae (arrowed) are present (note that the large
unstained negative area marked 'C' is a cyst within the tumor
and not a region of antigen-negative cells). (b): a higher
magnification view of the area outlined in (a) reveals one of
the negative regions (asterisk) in greater detail. The characteristic normal pattern of transferrin receptor expression
in squamous epithelium (i.e., staining confined to basal
layers) is seen in the overlying epidermis (arrowed).

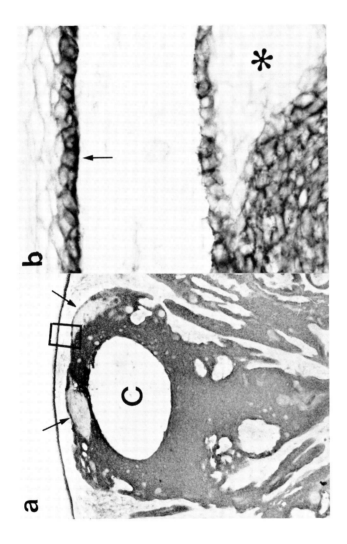

antigens and carcinoembryonic antigen. For some reason, lymphoid neoplasms appear to show this phenomenon much less frequently.

In a proportion of tumors, antigenic heterogeneity appears to be a reflection of localized differentiation occurring within the neoplasm, as illustrated in Figure 2. In other cases, however, no such process can be identified by conventional histological examination (Figure 3).

Thus, no comprehensive explanation exists for the heterogeneity of antigenic expression by many human epithelial neoplasms. We have observed that nonneoplastic epithelial tissue (e.g., the uterine cervix) may on occasion show a strikingly patchy expression of certain antigens (e.g., keratin-associated components) despite the fact that the tissue appears histologically homogeneous. Hence, the phenomenon may not be specific for neoplasia, but may indicate that non-neoplastic epithelial tissues exhibit more extensive cell-to-cell antigenic variation than has previously been suspected. Whatever its explanation, this irregular expression of antigens by human tumors has obvious implications for attempts to eradicate tumors using monoclonal antibodies complexed with drugs, toxins, isotopes, etc. Furthermore, studies which seek to relate the expression of an individual antigen (e.g., HLA-DR) to clinical features such as tumor growth and metastasis should take this phenomenon into account, since it may result in two samples taken from the same tumor giving different immunohistological labeling results.

B. 'Inappropriate' Antigen Expression

On occasion, epithelial tumors express antigens which are not present on the normal tissue from which they have arisen. However, testing of normal tissue of other types (e.g., other classes of epithelium) reveals that the antigens are found elsewhere in the body. The phenomenon is illustrated in Figure 4.

The wider implication of this phenomenon is that new monoclonal antibodies which appear to be specific for neoplastic cells should be tested extensively on a wide range of tissues by immunohistological techniques. To the best of the authors' knowledge, no monoclonal antibodies described to date have proven truly tumor- or neoplasia-specific when analyzed in this way.

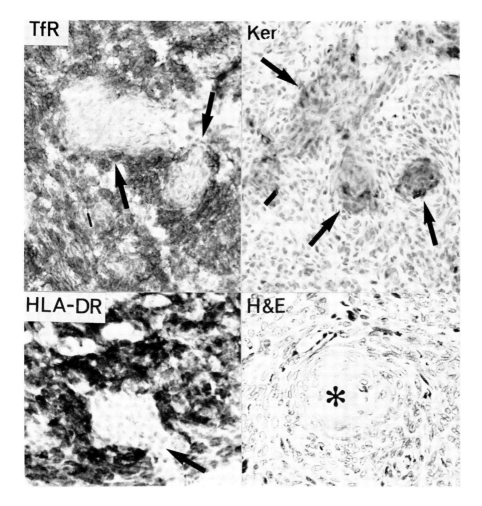

FIGURE 2. Immunoperoxidase staining of a cutaneous basal
cell carcinoma. Both transferrin receptor (TfR) and HLA-DR
show a similar labeling pattern of occasional negative areas
(arrowed), often rounded in outline, scattered against a background of positively stained cells. The reverse pattern is
observed when staining for a keratin-associated antigen (Ker),
suggesting that localized areas of squamous differentiation
(arrowed) account for the loss of TfR and HLA-DR. In fact,
such 'squamous eddies' could be seen (asterisk) in convention-
ally stained paraffin-embedded tissue from the same case (H
and E).

C. Diagnostic Applications of Monoclonal Antibodies

Diagnostic pathologists are regularly confronted by two problems of clinical relevance (resolution of which may significantly alter patient management). Firstly, they are often called upon to decide whether or not a tissue is neoplastic. Secondly, they frequently have to identify the cellular origin of a tumor (e.g., to distinguish between lymphoma and carcinoma, etc.).

Many laboratories have endeavored to produce monoclonal antibodies which will answer the first type of question; their enthusiasm apparently has been undampened by the generally negative outcome of attempts to find such markers by other means in the past. So far, the search for neoplasia-specific monoclonal antibodies has met with equally little success. Even when promising monoclonal antibodies of this type emerge in the future, the task of proving their reliability for the detection of tumor cells in tissue sections may pose considerable problems. This is because the interest of such antibodies will be centered primarily on their ability to detect early epithelial malignancy (e.g., to confirm suspected carcinoma in situ); however, when analyzing such lesions by immunohistological methods the pathologist will in effect be attempting to solve an equation in which there are two unknown values (i.e., the specificity of the antibody for malignant change, and the true nature of the suspect lesion).

The use of monoclonal antibodies to resolve the second type of diagnostic dilemma faced by pathologists (i.e., the identification of the cellular origin of tumors) has attracted less attention than the search for neoplasia-specific reagents. Nevertheless, a quiet revolution has taken place in this field since the first monoclonal antibodies against human tissues were produced. It is now possible, as detailed in previous publications from the authors' laboratory and other centers (1,2,3), to distinguish with certainty between poorly differentiated carcinoma and 'high grade' lymphoma - a frequent diagnostic problem in routine histopathology. The most valuable antigenic markers for this purpose are the leukocyte-common antigen (present on lymphoma cells) and several epithelia-associated antigens (present on carcinoma cells). Less work has been performed on identifying other types of anaplastic tumors, but the existence of monoclonal antibodies reactive with constituents such as desmin, vimentin, glial fibrillary acidic protein, neuroblastoma antigens, S-100 protein, etc., offers obvious promise in this direction.

There is one major practical obstacle, however, which restricts the application of such techniques in routine histopathological diagnosis. This is the fact that many of these

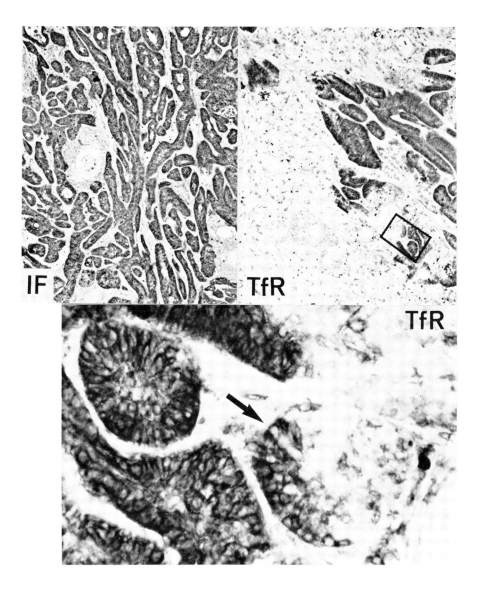

FIGURE 3. (upper): Adjacent sections from a uterine
adenocarcinoma stained by the immunoperoxidase technique for a
cytokeratin intermediate filament determinant (IF) and for
transferrin receptor (TfR). The anti-intermediate filament
antibody reacts with all of the neoplastic glandular tissue,
while TfR is only patchily expressed. The outlined area on
the section stained for TfR is shown at higher magnification
in the illustration below. Note that one acinus (arrowed)
seen in cross-section is divided approximately equally into
positive and negative areas.

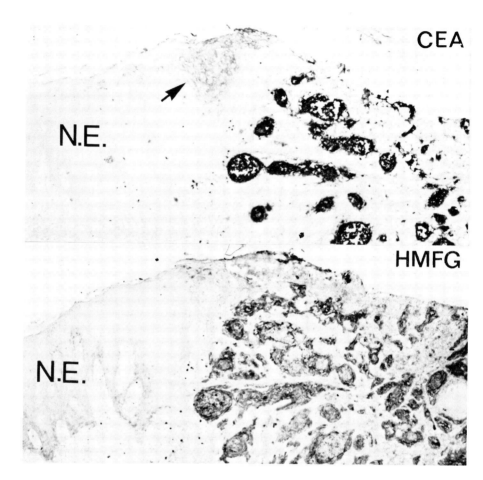

FIGURE 4. Squamous cell carcinoma of skin stained for carcinoembryonic antigen (CEA) and for human milk fat globule antigen (HMFG). Both constitutents are strongly expressed by the neoplastic cells, but are absent from the adjacent normal epithelium (N.E.). Within the restricted context of this sample, these antigens appear to be neoplasia-specific. When other tissues are stained, however, it is evident that they are widely distributed on nonsquamous epithelium. Note that there is weak focal expression (arrowed) of CEA on nonneoplastic epithelium close to the tumor.

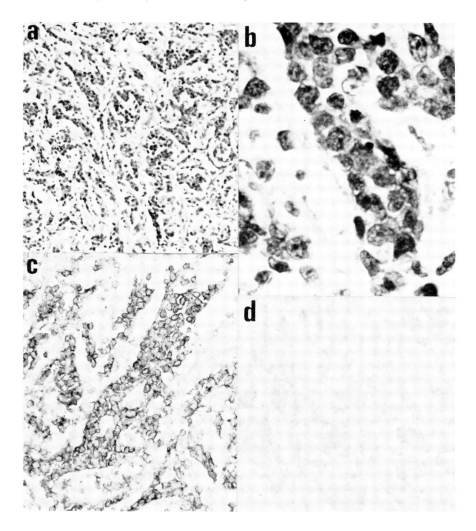

FIGURE 5. These photomicrographs illustrate the use of
the monoclonal anti-leukocyte antibody 2B11 for diagnosing
poorly differentiated lymphoid neoplasms in routine paraffin-
embedded biopsies. Conventional staining of this case
(a and b) revealed an anaplastic tumor which was diagnosed
independently by three different pathologists as a carcinoma.
In particular, the tendency of the tumor cells to grow in
sheets and cords, seen in high power in (b), was considered
typical of this type of tumor. However, immunoperoxidase
staining of paraffin sections with antibody 2B11 revealed
strong labeling of the tumor cells (c), and the diagnosis was
revised to one of lymphoma. The negative reaction of the
tumor with an anti-epithelial antibody (HMFG) is shown in (d).

monoclonal antibodies (particularly those directed against lymphoid cells) react with antigenic determinants which do not survive tissue fixation and paraffin embedding. The authors have, therefore, systematically evaluated a wide range of new monoclonal antibodies in an effort to find reagents which are not subject to this limitation. Recently, this has enabled us to identify two new monoclonal antibodies (PD7/26 and 2B11) both of which react with epitopes on the leukocyte-common molecule which are resistant to tissue processing (4).

Evaluation of these antibodies on a series of routine histological biopsies has shown that they can be relied upon to identify lymphoma cells in this type of material (Figure 5), and they are now used in the authors' laboratory and elsewhere for the routine diagnosis of poorly differentiated tumors. As the number of additional monoclonal antibodies which give satisfactory reactions with paraffin-embedded material increases, the scope of this approach to diagnosis will grow.

ACKNOWLEDGMENTS

We are grateful to the following collaborators for providing samples of antibodies: Drs. Joyce Taylor-Papadimitriou (HMFG2), E. B. Lane (LE61), G. Brown (BK19.9), C. Woodhouse and J. Corvalan (anti-CEA).

REFERENCES

1. Gatter, K.C., Abdulaziz, Z., Beverley, P., Corvalan, J.R.F., Ford, C., Lane, E.B., Mota, M., Nash, J.R.G., Pulford, K., Stein, H., Taylor-Papadimitriou, J., Woodhouse, C., and Mason, D.Y. J. Clin. Pathol. 35, 1253 (1982).
2. Pizzolo, G., Sloane, J., Beverley, P., Thomas, J.A., Bradstock, K.F., Mattingly, S. and Janossy, G. Cancer 46, 2640 (1980).
3. Battifora, H. and Trowbridge, I.S. Cancer 51, 816 (1983).
4. Warnke, R.A., Gatter, K.C., Falini, B., Hildreth, P., Woolston, R-E., Pulford, K., Cordell, J.L., Cohen, B., Wolf-Peeters, C. de. and Mason, D.Y. (Submitted for publication) (1983).

QUESTIONS AND ANSWERS

RIETHMÜLLER: Why are infiltrating lymphocytes negative for transferrin receptors?

MASON: T cells and macrophages could not be easily disting- uished in sections and we do know that transferrin receptors are well expressed on macrophages. Thus, at present we would guess that lymphocytes are probably negative in this situa- tion.

WOLF: Have you had any experience in the utilization of HLA- DR antibodies in the differentiation of melanoma from Nevi?

MASON: We have not looked at that yet.

WOLF: Do you believe that anti-keratin antibodies are useful to differentiate lymphomas from thymomas?

MASON: Yes, in each of three thymomas there was a very different, even bizarre, reaction pattern, although the epithelial components could be distinguished, with the anti-keratin antibodies.

LENNOX: A possible explanation for erratic expression of an antigenic determinant is that the determinant is association dependent.   There are examples of this with the transferrin receptor.

MASON: The problem here is that we are analyzing such complex structures as the cell surface with a single technique and it is hard to know when one is being distracted by potentially trivial explanations as opposed to major ones.

OSPINA: Can transferrin receptors be used in the study and classification of uterine cervical dysplasias?

MASON: In one study where we tried to follow this, we could not make any real distinctions.

MACH: You mentioned a monoclonal antibody against inter- mediary filament proteins.   What is the molecular weight of the antigen recognized?   Is it present in fibroblasts and glial cells?   Does it react with vimentin?

MASON: Perhaps I could ask Joyce to comment on this question.

TAYLOR-PAPADIMITRIOU: Comment - LE61 is a monoclonal antibody directed to one of the smaller MW cytokeratins (52K, in this case) and it is found only in simple nonkeratinizing epithelium. It does not react with other types of intermediate filaments.

Question — You said that LE61 does not stain squamous carcinoma, but sometimes HMFG-2 does. Does this hold for cervical epithelium? Does typically malignant cervical squamous epithelium show the same pattern of reaction with LE61 and HMFG-2 as described for skin?

MASON: Yes. LE61 does not stain normal cervical epithelium, but does stain occasional cells in malignancies.

SUN: Is the absence of IgM staining in lymphoid follicles good enough to be diagnostic for B cell malignancy?

MASON: Yes. This is very good evidence that it is neoplastic. In fact, it is a good example of how normal antigens can serve as markers for neoplasia.

DIFFERENTIAL REACTIVITY OF MONOCLONAL ANTIBODIES WITH HUMAN COLON ADENOCARCINOMAS AND ADENOMAS

Daniela Stramignoni, Robert Bowen and Jeffrey Schlom

Laboratory of Tumor Immunology and Biology
National Cancer Institute
National Institutes of Health
Bethesda, Maryland

Barbara F. Atkinson

Department of Pathology and Laboratory Medicine
University of Pennsylvania
Philadelphia, Pennsylvania

I. INTRODUCTION

Monoclonal antibodies to human colon, lung and breast carcinomas have been generated in a number of laboratories. A surprising finding of these studies has been the large number of antigenic cross-reactivities observed among these three major carcinoma groups. We have recently generated a series of monoclonal antibodies (including B72.3 and B6.2) using membrane-enriched fractions of human metastatic mammary carcinomas as immunogen (1). B72.3 is reactive with a 220,000d-400,000d high molecular weight glycoprotein complex, while B6.2 is reactive with a 90,000d glycoprotein. We have also used membrane-enriched fractions of human metastatic mammary carcinomas to generate two monoclonal antibodies (B1.1 and F5.5) that are reactive with purified carcinoembryonic antigen (CEA) from colon carcinoma patients. Both B1.1 and F5.5 immunoprecipitate the characteristic 180,000d CEA glycoprotein (2).

Monoclonal antibody B72.3 reacts with tissue sections of approximately 50% of human breast carcinomas, while B6.2 and B1.1 react with approximately 75-80% of these lesions (3,4). None react appreciably with adjacent normal mammary tissue, nor with the surface of approximately twenty-five normal human cell lines tested. Monoclonal antibodies B1.1 (anti-CEA) and B6.2 have shown a great deal of coordinate expression on the surface of many of the tumor lines and tumor tissue samples tested; they also have shown reactivities to polymorphonuclear leukocytes and sweat glands in tissue sections. Monoclonal antibody B72.3, on the other hand, has shown no appreciable reactivity to any normal human cell line, normal tissue sections, or normal extracts tested. Monoclonal antibodies B72.3, B1.1 and B6.2 have shown no reactivity to the surface of sarcoma cell lines or hematopoetic malignancies. The studies reported here were designed to define the range of reactivities of monoclonal antibodies B72.3, B6.2 and B1.1 to colon adenocarcinomas and adenomas versus benign colon lesions and normal colon epithelium.

II. RESULTS

Purified IgG of monoclonal antibody B1.1 was reacted with fixed, 5 micron tissue sections of malignant and benign colon lesions at concentrations of 10, 1 and 0.1µg of purified IgG per slide using the avidin-biotin complex (ABC) method of immunoperoxidase staining. The characteristic dark reddish-brown positive reaction was contrasted with that of the blue hematoxylin counterstain. Scoring of carcinomas was based on the percentage of positive carcinoma cells as well as the intensity of the stain. Using 10µg/ml of B1.1, 94% (15 of 16) of colon carcinomas from different patients scored positive (Figure 1A). All the positive carcinomas contained more than 25% reactive cells; in three of the tumors, 100% of the cells were positive. A heterogeneity of antigenic expression in terms of lumenal versus cytoplasmic reactivity in a given tumor mass was usually observed. Approximately two-thirds of coexistent adenoma lesions and normal colon epithelium also were positive (Figure 1A). The majority of adenomas from noncarcinoma patients (Figure 1A) and one of two diverticul-itis specimens also scored positive. Using lower dilutions of B1.1 (1µg/ml and 0.1µg/ml), the majority of colon carcinoma specimens remained positive. Some of the adenomas in non-carcinoma patients also remained positive, scoring from 71% positive using 1µg/ml to 44% positive using 0.1µg/ml of B1.1.

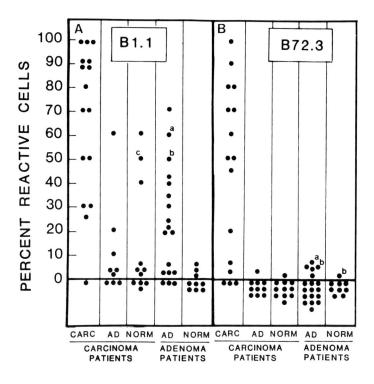

FIGURE 1.   Scoring of immunoperoxidase staining with monoclonal antibody B1.1 (A), and B72.3 (B) (both at 10µg/ml).
The first three columns of Panels A and B show the reactivity
of carcinomas (CARC), adenomas (AD) and normal epithelium
(NORM) in carcinoma-bearing patients.   The next two columns
show the reactivity of adenomas (AD) and normal epithelium
(NORM) in adenoma-bearing patients.   (a) Tubular adenoma in a
patient with 'probable recurrence' of colon carcinoma.
(b) Tubulovillous adenoma with atypia and diagnosis of in situ
carcinoma.   (c) Colon cancer patient with ulcerative colitis.

Using 10μg/ml of monoclonal antibody B72.3, 14 of 17 (82%) of colon carcinomas demonstrated a variable number of positive staining cells (Figure 1B). The majority of the carcinomas that were positive had more than 50% of tumor cells reacting. Only two of the 14 positive samples had 5% or less of the tumor cells reacting. In only one of the 17 carcinomas tested, did 100% of tumor cells react with B72.3. In all other positive samples, varying degrees of antigenic hetero-geneity of a given tumor mass were observed. Strongly reactive cells have been seen adjacent to negative cells. The cellular location of the reactivity also varied within a given tumor mass. Lumenal reactivity was often observed in glandu-lar structures, while cytoplasmic staining was observed in less differentiated structures. In a few cases, focal stain-ing of cytoplasmic structures and intracellular vacuolar staining were also observed. Parallel slides with phosphate-buffered saline (instead of primary antibody B72.3), isotype-identical IgG (MOPC-21), as well as normal murine IgG were used as controls for the specificity of the staining observed. All of these gave negative results.

Adenomas in patients with colon carcinoma were also examined for expression of antigen reactive with monoclonal antibody B72.3. Only one of ten such lesions showed a posi-tive reaction (Figure 1B). This lesion was immediately adja-cent to a carcinoma and had less than 5% cells positive. All other adenomas and adjacent normal epithelium in carcinoma patients were negative, with one exception in which less than 1% of the cells scored positive.

Adenomas from patients without apparent carcinoma were examined using 10μg/ml monoclonal antibody B72.3. Five of the 18 samples showed staining in a few percent of adenoma cells (Figure 1B). Sections of normal colon epithelium adjacent to adenomas from nine patients examined showed no reactivity to monoclonal antibody B72.3, except for a patient in which less than one percent of normal epithelium showed reactivity. None of the samples of three patients with diverticulitis showed any reactivity with monoclonal antibody B72.3.

Malignant and benign lesions were then examined using ten-fold less (1μg/ml) monoclonal antibody B72.3. At this antibody dilution, 50% (8/16) of carcinomas showed a positive reaction; one of ten adjacent adenomas showed a focal reactivity of less than one percent of adenomatous cells. None of 16 adenomas from noncarcinoma patients and none of 19 normal epithelia from carcinoma or adenoma patients reacted at this antibody dilution. Thus, a positive reactivity with monoclonal antibody B72.3 at this dilution appears to be an even stronger marker for malignancy.

As mentioned above, monoclonal antibodies B1.1 and B6.2 can be distinguished on the basis of the molecular weight of the proteins precipitated from tumor cells. From reactivity patterns on tumor and normal tissues, it has been difficult thus far to distinguish the reactivities of these two monoclonal antibodies. Used at 10μg/ml, monoclonal antibody B6.2 reacted with all of 15 colon carcinomas tested, with three of the tumors showing 100% reactivity. Three of ten adenomas, as well as two of eleven normal epithelia, adjacent to carcinoma lesions were positive. Using 10μg/ml of B6.2 per slide, 65% (11/17) of adenomas from noncarcinoma patients also scored positive as did one of two diverticulitis lesions.

Using 1μg/ml of monoclonal antibody B6.2 per slide, 93% (14/15) of carcinoma lesions scored positive. Two of ten adenomas in carcinoma patients and 30% (5/16) of adenomas from noncarcinoma patients also were positive. However, with the exception of one lesion, all adenomas had less than ten percent tumor cells positive. Using 0.1μg/ml of B6.2, 8/15 carcinomas were positive while three of eighteen adenomas were positive with only a few percent of cells reacting. Thus, monoclonal antibody B6.2 was clearly different from monoclonal antibody B1.1, because it was more selective towards colon carcinoma versus adenomas or normal colon epithelium. The reactivity of B6.2, however, was not as selective for carcinomas as was that observed for monoclonal antibody B72.3.

Seven cases of ulcerative colitis were examined with the three monoclonal antibodies at 10μg/ml. Focal positivity was observed with monoclonal antibody 72.3 in three of seven cases. The three positive cases all had an active inflammatory infiltrate and architectural glandular atypia, whereas the negative cases did not. Two of seven, and four of seven lesions were positive with monoclonal antibodies B1.1 and B6.2, respectively. The percent of cells reactive varied with each sample, from less than 5% to greater than 30%.

Fourteen colon carcinomas were 'phenotyped' on the basis of their expression of the antigens reactive with monoclonal antibodies B72.3, B6.2 and B1.1. When all the monoclonal antibodies are used at 10μg/ml, only one major phenotype (containing 13 of 14 lesions) emerges, i.e., the phenotype showing reactivity with all the monoclonal antibodies. When the monoclonal antibodies are all used at 1μg/ml, however, five phenotypes emerge; when monoclonal antibodies are used at 0.1μg/ml still a different phenotypic pattern emerges. It thus appears from these studies that one can group or phenotype colon carcinomas on the basis of their degree of differential expression of specific tumor-associated antigens. Using the higher concentrations of monoclonal antibodies may not be the best for making distinctions, i.e., distinguishing

a tumor expressing high levels of antigen versus one
expressing low levels.

Colon adenomas were also phenotyped in a similar manner;
four distinct antigenic phenotypes are observed using 10µg/ml.
When using 1µg/ml of monoclonal antibodies, the distribution
of tumors within a given group is changed. The biologic significance of a given phenotype for a carcinoma or adenoma
lesion remains to be determined.

III. DISCUSSION

Numerous studies have been reported on the use of immunohistochemical methods to detect CEA in tissue sections of
colon carcinomas and normal colon epithelium. As mentioned
previously, however, the results reported vary for almost
every study. The use of monoclonal antibodies should help
greatly in both standardizing results and comparing findings
between laboratories. The results reported above demonstrate
the importance of the titer of immunoglobulin used in interpretation of results. Atkinson et al. (5) have reported on
the reactivity of a monoclonal antibody (19-9) against a mono-
ganglioside antigen associated with colon carcinomas. This
antigen is present in 59% of colon carcinomas. The presentation of this antigen in colon lesions is clearly distinct from
any of the antigens detected in this study. Various tumors,
as well as areas within a given tumor, show a discordance of
reactivity between monoclonal antibody 19-9 and monoclonal
antibodies B1.1, B6.2 and B72.3 (B. Atkinson, personal observations).

The most selective reactivity for colon carcinomas versus
benign tumors and normal tissues was observed with monoclonal
antibody B72.3. The 220,000d-400,000d glycoprotein complex
detected by this antigen appears to be a novel tumor-
associated antigen. While similarly sized glycoproteins have
been previously reported present in melanomas (6-8), monoclonal antibody B72.3 shows no reactivity to this class of
tumors.

On the basis of the selective reactivity of B72.3 for
malignant and atypical lesions, this marker may eventually be
useful as an indicator of malignant change in histologic and
cytologic material. This may be particularly useful in the
examination of patients with an increased risk for development
of carcinoma. For this reason we examined biopsies of seven
patients with ulcerative colitis. This disease carries a 5-11
times greater risk, compared to the normal population (1 in

20), for developing colorectal cancer. In three of seven of these cases, positive reactions were observed only when archi-tectural glandular atypia and active inflammation were present. These results indicate that ulcerative colitis patients can be divided into positive- and negative-reacting categories. The significance of this classification in regards to malignant propensity requires further study.

In summary, colon carcinomas, adenomas, and ulcerative colitis can now be antigenically phenotyped into several dis-tinct groups based on their reactivity with the three mono-clonal antibodies employed in this study. Large retrospective studies using fixed tissue sections can now be conducted to determine if a given antigenic phenotype correlates with a specific biologic property such as response to a specific therapeutic modality or prognosis.

ABBREVIATIONS

CEA, carcinoembryonic antigen.

REFERENCES

1. Colcher, D., Horan Hand, P., Nuti, M. and Schlom, J. Proc. Natl. Acad. Sci. USA 78, 3199 (1981).
2. Colcher, D., Horan Hand, P., Nuti, M. and Schlom, J. Cancer Invest. 1, 131 (1983).
3. Nuti, M, Teramoto, Y.A., Mariani-Constantini, R., Horan Hand, P., Colcher, D. and Schlom, J. Int. J. Cancer 29, 539 (1982).
4. Horan Hand, P., Nuti, M., Colcher, D. and Schlom, J. Cancer Res. 43, 728 (1983).
5. Atkinson, B.F., Ernst, C.S., Herlyn, M., Steplewski, Z., Sears, H.F. and Koprowski, H. Cancer Res. 42, 4820 (1982).
6. Mitchell, K.F., Fuhrer, J.P., Steplewski, Z. and Koprowski, H. Proc. Natl. Acad. Sci. USA 77, 7287 (1980).
7. Loop, S.M., Hellstrom, I., Woodbury, RC., Brown, J.P. and Hellstrom, K.E. Int. J. Cancer 27, 775 (1981).
8. Wilson, B.S, Kohzoh, I, Natali, P.G and Ferrone, S. Int. J. Cancer 28, 293 (1981).

QUESTIONS AND ANSWERS

LENNOX: As a point of clarification, is B72.3 directed against CEA?

SCHLOM: No. B72.3 has nothing to do with CEA. It is not coordinately expressed. The molecular weights of the proteins are very different, etc. The only thing in common is that it does react with other carcinomas.

DULBECCO: Was there reactivity with the colon in the ulcerative colitis slide?

SCHLOM: No, but there is shedding of the antigen in a lot of these cases.

DULBECCO: How do you know?

SCHLOM: We see it in the blood.

McGEE: Regarding the B72.3 staining, how long did your patients have ulcerative colitis?

SCHLOM: I just do not know. This is a case where we must do a good retrospective study, going back 20–30 years.

MONOCLONAL ANTIBODIES POTENTIALLY USEFUL IN CLINICAL ONCOLOGY[1]

Maria Ines Colnaghi, Silvana Canevari,
Gabriella Della Torre, Sylvie Mènard, Silvia Miotti,
Mario Regazzoni and Elda Tagliabue

Division of Experimental Oncology A
Istituto Nazionale Tumori
Milano, Italy

Renato Mariani-Costantini and Franco Rilke

Division of Anatomical Pathology and Cytology
Istituto Nazionale Tumori
Milano, Italy

I. MATERIALS AND METHODS

The technique we have used for hybridoma production and the screening methodologies we have used for identification of monoclonal reagents suitable for clinical applications already have been described (1-4). The material used in defining the specificity of our monoclonal reagents is listed in Table 1. We identified three monoclonal antibodies which appear promising. MBr1 (IgM) was obtained from immunization against human breast cancer cells; MOv1 and MOv2 (IgG1 and IgM, respectively) were obtained from immunization with human ovarian cancer cells. MBr1, which recognizes a cell membrane neutral glycolipid antigen, was found to react against about

---

[1]This work was partially supported by a grant from Consiglio Nazionale delle Ricerche, Rome, Italy (Progetto Finalizzato Controllo della Crescita Neoplastica, Contract No. 81.01387.96).

80% of ductal, lobular and tubular breast cancers, whereas it was found to be negative on colloid and papillary carcinomas and breast carcinoids. Among the cell lines and the normal tissues listed in Table 1, MBr1 was found to react with two breast cancer cell lines, mammary duct epithelial cells, some distal and collecting tubules of kidney and some epithelia of the genital system; in addition, a focal labeling was found in exocrine pancreas, sweat and salivary glands. MOv1, which recognizes a high MW glycoprotein secreted by ovarian cells, was found to react with 100% of mucinous ovarian tumors tested; whereas it was found to be negative on all cell lines tested. Among normal tissues, MOv1 was found to react with intestinal glands only. MOv2, which recognizes a high MW membrane glycoprotein, was found to react with 70% of ovarian carcinomas of various histological types and 40% of other carcinomas; whereas, among the normal tissues, it was found to react with digestive tract glands and lactating mammary ducts. All other lines, normal tissues, tumors and proteins listed in Table 1 were negative with the three monoclonals.

II. RESULTS

Because MBr1 detects both primary and metastatic tumor cells, we have tested its ability to discriminate breast cancer cells from normal cells in bone marrow samples from patients with a previous history of breast cancer. Thirty-nine bone marrow samples were examined. The results obtained by conventional histology were compared to those obtained by immunofluorescence (IF) with MBr1. In seventeen cases, a bone marrow involvement was diagnosed by conventional histology and confirmed by positive IF with MBr1. Of twenty-two cases that scored negative by conventional histology, seven scored positive by IF. As controls, numerous bone marrow samples from nontumor patients or patients with nonbreast tumors were examined; no positive cells were found in any case. It seems, therefore, that the use of the MBr1 monoclonal antibody may improve the conventional diagnostic procedures employed to detect micrometastases in the bone marrow.

We considered the possibility of applying our monoclonal antibodies as an improved tool in cytopathological diagnosis. First of all we ascertained their reactivities on nonneoplastic cells which can be present in body fluids. We used pleural and peritoneal effusions from noncancer patients and from patients with cancer other than that of breast and

TABLE 1.   Material Used in Defining the Specificity of
Monoclonal Antibodies

Cell Lines

Carcinoma: Breast (MCF-7, SK-BR-3)
                        Ovary (SW 626), Stomach (KATO III)
                        Colon (HT-29), Bladder (VM-CUB-3)
                        Kidney (A498, A704)

Sarcoma: (SaOS, SW 684)

Melanoma: (MeWo, Me20, Me9556)

Lymphoid Cells: (Daudi)

Normal Tissues and Corresponding Tumors (Surgical specimens)

Kidney, urinary bladder, prostate, liver, gall bladder, lung,
larynx, stomach, pancreas, large and small intestine, ovary,
uterus, testis, skin, sweat glands, sebaceous glands, mammary
glands, adrenal glands, salivary glands, thyroid, muscle, bone
marrow, leukocytes, spleen, thymus, red blood cells, nervous
tissue

Proteins

Fetal calf serum, human plasma, total milk proteins, casein,
lactoferrin, whey proteins

---

ovary. When tested by direct IF with MBr1 and MOv2 monoclonal
antibodies, there was no labeling of cells of any type,
irrespective of whether the effusions were positive or
negative cytologically.
     We then examined twenty-five pleural effusions from breast
cancer patients and forty-one peritoneal effusions from ovary
cancer patients. We used both conventional cytology and IF
with MBr1 and MOv2 monoclonal antibodies. The results are
given in Table 2.
     In order to identify the type of labeled cells, an
electron microscopic immunoperoxidase test was carried out on
cells from effusions that were cytopathologically positive for

metastatic breast or ovary carcinoma cells and also positive
in IF with the relevant monoclonal antibody. The results
obtained confirmed that the labeled cells were mammary or
ovary epithelial tumor cells. Mesothelial cells, as well as
polymorphonuclear leukocytes, lymphocytes and red blood cells
(clearly identified ultrastructurally) were always negative
(Figure 1).

TABLE 2. Reactivity of MBr1 and MOv2 Monoclonal
Antibodies With Cells From Twenty-Five Pleural
Effusions of Breast Cancer Patients and
Forty-One Peritoneal Effusions of Ovarian
Carcinoma Patients

Number of Cases	Cytological Diagnosis	IF Number of Positive Cases/ Total Tested Cases	
		MBr1	MOv2
Breast Cancer			
25 pleural	10 negative	0/10	ND
Effusions	11 positive	8/11	ND
Examined	4 negative	4/4	ND
Ovarian Cancer			
41 peritoneal	21 negative	0/21	0/16
Effusions	17 positive	10/17	6/16
Examined	3 negative	3/3	2/3

ND = not done

The results of Table 2 show that among the breast cancer
patients ten effusions were negative by both cytology and IF
with MBr1. Among eleven effusions cytopathologically
diagnosed as positive, only eight were found to have cells
positive with MBr1. The negativity of the other three cases
may be due to the fact that MBr1 reacts with about 80% of the
most common types of breast cancer. Four cases were found
negative by cytological examination but positive in IF by
MBr1. The positivity was confirmed by further clinical,
pathological and electron microscopic examinations. These

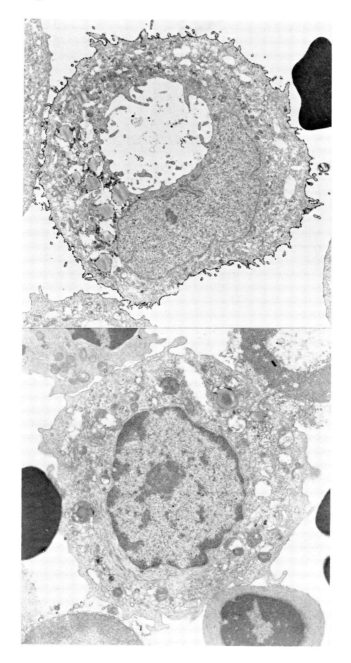

FIGURE 1. Immunoperoxidase electron microscopy with MBr1
monoclonal antibody: A) Specific surface labeling of a breast
cancer cell showing an intracytoplasmic lumen (x6,400). B) A
mesothelial cell, showing perinuclear bundles of filaments,
completely unlabeled (x13,400).

data indicate that the use of MBr1 in IF cannot at present substitute for the conventional diagnostic procedure, but is helpful in reducing the proportion of false negative cases.

With regard to ovarian cancer, the IF test was carried out with MOv2 and in parallel with MBr1 monoclonal antibody, because the latter was shown to react with about 40% of the ovarian carcinomas. This was done to see whether the detection of cancer cells increased using two reagents which probably recognize different epitopes on the cells of a given type of tumor. Twenty-one cytopathologically negative cases also were found negative by IF with both monoclonal antibodies. Among the seventeen cytopathologically positive cases, ten scored positive by IF with MBr1 and six with MOv2, for a total of thirteen positive cases. Therefore, the simultaneous use of two reagents was found to improve the diagnostic efficiency. Three cytopathologically negative cases were found positive by IF; the positivity was confirmed by further clinical and pathological examination. We expect that the availability of a library of monoclonal antibodies directed against different epitopes of tumor cells may afford in the near future new, more sensitive methodologies for cytopathological diagnosis.

In addition, the anti-ovarian carcinoma MOv1 monoclonal antibody, which recognizes a secretion product of the ovarian cells, is being studied to ascertain whether it can detect the relevant antigen in circulation by radioimmunoassay (RIA). A

TABLE 3.   Detection of MOv1-Recognized Antigen in Plasma and Peritoneal Fluid by Solid-Phase RIA

	Ovarian Cancer Patients	Patients With Other Tumors	Healthy Subjects and Non-Cancer Patients
MOv1 positive*/ total tested cases	11/22	4/15	0/13
Antigen concentration in positive cases	94.8ng/ml	36.2ng/ml	–
Antigen concentration in negative cases	9.3ng/ml	6.3ng/ml	3.1ng/ml

* Positivity = >30ng/ml

solid-phase immunoradiometric assay was employed in which the
purified antigen, obtained from a surgical specimen of a
mucinous ovarian carcinoma, was attached to the microplate
wells and then reacted with ^{125}I-labeled MOv1 monoclonal
antibody. A standard curve was obtained by inhibition of the
reaction wtih the same purified and solubilized antigen. The
cut-off was established at 30ng/ml.

In preliminary study, fifty ascites fluids or plasma from
patients with ovary and nonovary cancer, as well as from
nontumor patients and normal individuals, were examined. As
shown in Table 3, the level of the antigen was elevated in 50%
of twenty-two ovarian tumor patients and in 26% of fifteen
patients with other types of cancers. None of thirteen
nontumor patients or normal individuals showed elevated
antigen levels.

ABBREVIATIONS

IF, immunofluorescence; RIA, radioimmunoassay.

REFERENCES

1. Colnaghi, M.I., Clemente, C., Della Porta, G., Della
    Torre, G., Mariani-Costantini, R., Mènard S., Rilke, F.,
    and Tagliabue, E.   In 'Monoclonal Antibodies '82:
    Progress and Perspectives' (F. Dammacco, G. Doria and
    A. Pinchera, eds.) p. 79-95.   Elsevier/North Holland
    Biomedical Press (1983).
2. Mariani-Costantini, R., Mènard, S., Clemente, C.,
    Tagliabue, E., Colnaghi, M.I., and Rilke, F. J. Clin.
    Pathol. 35, 1037 (1982).
3. Canevari, S., Fossati, G., Balsari, A., Sonnino, S., and
    Colnaghi, M.I. Cancer Res. 43, 1301 (1983).
4. Mènard, S., Tagliabue, E., Canevari, S., Fossati, G. and
    Colnaghi, M.I. Cancer Res. 43, 1295 (1983).

CLINICAL SIGNIFICANCE OF THE MONOCLONAL ANTIBODY
ANTI-Y 29/55, REACTIVE AGAINST HUMAN FOLLICULAR
CENTER-DERIVED B LYMPHOCYTES AND THEIR
NEOPLASTIC COUNTERPARTS

Hansjörg K. Forster and Theo Staehelin

Central Research Units
F. Hoffmann-La Roche and Co. Ltd.
Basel, Switzerland

Jean-Paul Obrecht

Department of Internal Medicine
University Clinics
Kantonal Hospital
Basel, Switzerland

Fred G. Gudat

Institute of Pathology
University of Basel
Basel, Switzerland

I. INTRODUCTION

The clinical application of monoclonal antibodies is best
understood in the context of the anatomy and pathology of the
target cells such antibodies recognize. The architecture of
lymphoid tissues has been reviewed by Weissman et al. (1).
Lymphoid follicles are the sites of B cell proliferation and
differentiation, particularly of antigen-inexperienced B lymphocytes. The production of functionally distinct B memory
cells and immunoglobulin-secreting plasma cells then proceeds

in this environment. However, B cell differentiation can
occur independently of antigenic stimulation, as has been
shown in germfree animals.

In man, the differentiation sequence of B lymphocytes in
follicular centers has been described by morphological
criteria (2). In a first step, the nucleus of small lymphocytes develops a cleaved shape. By gradual enlargement and
acquisition of a small amount of cytoplasm, a second stage is
reached, the large cleaved follicular center cell. In further
stages the nucleus rounds up and a small nucleolus appears;
and, later, abundant cytoplasm and one to three more prominent
nucleoli develop, often situated on the nuclear membrane (cen-
troblast) (3). The cleaved cells of the follicular center
are, for the most part, nondividing, whereas all of the noncleaved cells are part of a proliferating population. The
large noncleaved cells develop to B immunoblasts and plasma
cells, and are then found in the interfollicular areas and
medullary cords of lymphoid tissues. Such resting and stimulated human B lymphocytes, normally confined to peripheral
lymphoid tissues like lymph nodes, spleen, and tonsils, exhibit a membrane component recognized by the monoclonal murine
antibody anti-Y 29/55 (4,5).

II. RESULTS

Anti-Y 29/55, which consists of γ2a and κ chains and binds
complement, was derived from a fusion between a γ1 heavy
chain-deficient mouse myeloma line and splenocytes of a mouse
immunized with peripheral blood lymphocytes from a patient
with untreated chronic lymphocytic leukemia of the B cell
type. Reactivity with a membrane component on target cells
was demonstrated by use of a microcytotoxicity assay or
indirect immunofluorescence (IF). The antigen recognized is
expressed on B lymphocytes along the maturation path to plasma
cell in secondary lymphoid organs. Anti-Y 29/55 still reacts
with B immunoblasts, but only weakly if at all with the
antibody-secreting plasma cell, as has been visualized by
electron microscopy after indirect immunoperoxidase
staining (6).

Lymphocyte subpopulations from peripheral blood of healthy
volunteers and of patients with reactive lymphocytosis or
nonleukemic multiple myeloma were not lysed by anti-Y 29/55.
Indirect IF studies on B lymphocyte-enriched populations of
normal peripheral blood, however, revealed a fraction (varying
between 0 and 40%)(7) that reacted with the antibody. In our

own laboratory, we never found this fraction to be more than
10%. B lymphocyte-enriched populations stimulated in vitro
with lectins or Epstein-Barr virus transformation did not
become reactive with this monoclonal antibody. The antibody
does not identify private or public histocompatibility markers
and membrane components common to recirculating lymphocytes
like surface Ig, enzymes, hormone receptors, Fc receptors,
structural proteins, etc. This conclusion is based on the
observation that normal peripheral blood lymphocyte populations of different histocompatibility phenotypes did not exhibit a common reactivity pattern.

Pathologically, neoplasms of the B cell compartment of the
immune system are B leukemias and B non-Hodgkin's lymphomas.
Anti-Y 29/55 reacts with the malignant lymphocyte populations
in peripheral blood of patients with B cell chronic lymphocytic leukemia (B-CLL), leukemic variant of B non-Hodgkin's
lymphoma (B-NHL), and hairy cell leukemia (HCL). Anti-Y 29/55
does not discriminate between differentiation steps within
this group; for instance, it does not separate B-CLL from well
differentiated lymphocytic lymphoma or HCL. It is important
to note that anti-Y 29/55 reacts with sessile B lymphocytes at
all stages of follicular differentiation within the secondary
lymphoid organs. These include the resting cells, committed
lymphocytes (as seen in the well differentiated lymphocyte of
B-CLL) and the large, undifferentiated blast (the neoplastic
counterpart of which is the transformed follicle center cell).
Lymphocytes of these differentiation stages are termed 'poorly
differentiated lymphocytes and/or histiocytes' in the lymphoma
nomenclature of Rappaport (8), 'small and/or large follicle
center cells' in the nomenclature of Lukes and Collins (2), or
'centrocytes and/or centroblasts' in the nomenclature of
Lennert (3).

The sequence proposed for the follicular center differentiation (2) parallels a development occasionally observed in
B cell lymphomas. A lymphoma that is initially a small
cleaved follicular center cell type with moderate malignancy
may later change to the highly aggressive noncleaved follicular center cell type (2). Thus, during progression of
lymphoid neoplasms, phenotypically different B cell
populations may develop and exist simultaneously. Such an
event was demonstrated in patients with B-CLL by use of the
fluorescence-activated cell sorter. Peripheral blood lymphocytes bound anti-Y 29/55 followed by F(ab')$_2$ rabbit anti-mouse
coupled to rhodamine. Three-dimensional distributions of cell
frequencies were established with respect to two independent
parameters, cell size and immunofluorescence intensity (9).

In some patients, the malignant cells consisted of at
least two populations differing in cell size and fluorescence

intensity. Several explanations are possible. Simultaneous neoplastic transformation events might have affected a number of cells differing in their state of maturation, leading to a stable plurifocal neoplasm. If the neoplastic transformation was monofocal, it is equally conceivable that during the progression of the leukemia further differentiation may have taken place, leading to subpopulations arrested at different stages of differentiation. These results demonstrate the broad spectrum of anti-Y 29/55 reactivity with human leukemic B lymphocytes derived from follicular center differentiation.

B lymphocytes populating secondary lymphoid organs are considered to arise ultimately from hematopoietic stem cells. In the fetus, B cells arise in the liver (reviewed by Melchers in 10). Postnatal B lymphopoiesis occurs in the bone marrow, which is the major repository of lymphoid stem cells. These cells are capable of reconstituting lymphoid organs. Even though complete information on the differentiation in bone marrow is not yet available, Figure 1 shows a tentative model.

Additional information comes from the study of human lymphoproliferative diseases. The cell phenotype seen in the common variant of acute lymphoblastic leukemia (ALL) is a putative B lineage progenitor (11). Primary B cell maturation in bone marrow comprises several steps whose neoplastic coun-terparts are null ALL, common ALL, pre-B ALL, and pre-B/B ALL. Cells of these neoplastic types showed no reactivity with anti-Y 29/55. No correlation could be found with any of the markers in ALL. It seems that early pre-B cell differen-tiation in bone marrow does not lead to expression of the antigen recognized by anti-Y 29/55 (12).

III. CONCLUSIONS

The diagnostic value of anti-Y 29/55 lies in the recog-nition of circulating leukemic cells in B-CLL, B-NHL, or HCL. In histological analysis, anti-Y 29/55 may serve to establish the B cell nature of tumors and distinguish these from T cell neoplasias or other large cell tumors, like undifferentiated leukemias or nonhematological tumors.

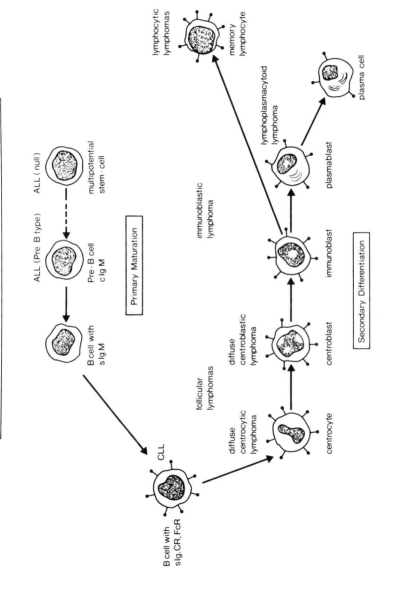

FIGURE 1. Expression of Y 29/55 antigen (🟡).

Elimination of malignant B lymphocyte populations from remission marrow might become a useful therapeutic application of anti-Y 29/55 in treatment of B-NHL. Subtypes of lymphomas like Burkitt's type B-NHL of stage IV (13) are still characterized by a very poor prognosis, even though increasingly aggressive cytotoxic regimens are successful in other pediatric lymphoid malignancies. Severe toxicity limits the intensity of therapeutic regimens. Hematopoietic reconstitution without tumor recurrence might be achieved by autologous bone marrow transplantation after extracorporeal treatment of isolated bone marrow cell suspensions. Anti-Y 29/55 might be efficient in bone marrow purging since it reacts with B cells of all differentiation steps past normal bone marrow maturation, thus leaving the cells required for lymphopoiesis unimpaired. Preliminary experience with this approach is presented elsewhere in this proceedings (14).

ABBREVIATIONS

IF, immunofluorescence; B-CLL, B cell chronic lymphocytic leukemia; B-NHL, B cell non-Hodgkin's lymphoma; HCL, hairy cell leukemia; ALL, acute lymphoblastic leukemia.

ACKNOWLEDGMENTS

The authors gratefully acknowledge the excellent technical contribution of Renate Albrecht, Manuela Deflorin and Marie-Françoise Girard.

REFERENCES

1. Weissman, I.L., Gutman, G.A. and Friedberg, S.G. Ser. Haematol. 7, 482 (1974).
2. Lukes, R.J., Parker, J.W., Taylor, C.R., Tindle, B.H., Cramer, A.D. and Lincoln, T.L. Ser. Haematol. 15, 322 (1978).
3. Lennert, K. In 'Malignant Lymphomas' (K. Lennert, ed.), p. 83. Springer-Verlag, Berlin (1978).

4. Forster, H.K., Gudat, F.G., Girard, M.F., Albrecht, R., Schmidt, J., Ludwig, C. and Obrecht, J.P. Cancer Res. 42, 1927 (1982).

5. Forster, H.K., Suter, F., Gudat, F.G. and Obrecht, J.P. In 'In Vivo Immunology' (P. Nieuwenhuis, A.A. van den Broek and M.G. Hanna, Jr., eds.), p. 61. Plenum Press, New York (1982).

6. Gudat, F.G., Forster, H.K., Girard, M.F., Albrecht, R., Ludwig, C. and Obrecht, J.P. In 'Leukemia Markers' (W. Knapp, ed.), p. 109. Academic Press, New York (1981).

7. Bernard, A. and Boumsell, L. In 'Human Leukocyte Markers Detected by Monoclonal Antibodies' (J. Dausset, C. Milstein and S.F. Schlossman, eds.) Springer-Verlag, Berlin (1983).

8. Rappaport, H. In 'Atlas of Tumor Pathology', Sect. 3, Fascicle 8. Armed Forces Institute of Pathology, Washington, D.C. (1966).

9. Forster, H.K., Obrecht, J.P., Knaak, T., Baumgartner, C., Wagner, H.P. and Gudat, F.G. In 'Human Leukocyte Markers Detected by Monoclonal Antibodies' (J. Dausset, C. Milstein and S.F. Schlossman, eds.) Springer-Verlag, Berlin (1983).

10. Melchers, F., von Boehmer, H., and Phillips, R.A. Transplant. Rev. 25, 26 (1975).

11. Greaves, M., Robinson, J., Delia, D., Sutherland, R., Newman, R. and Sieff, C. In 'Microenviromments in Haemopoietic and Lymphoid Differentiation' (Ciba Foundation Symposium 84), p. 109. Pitman, London (1981).

12. Hirt, A., Baumgartner, C., Forster, H.K., Imbach, P. and Wagner, H.P., Cancer Research (in press) (1983).

13. Grogan, T.M., Warnke, R.A. and Kaplan, H.S. Cancer 49, 1817 (1982).

14. Baumgartner, C., Imbach, P., Luthy, A., Odavic, R. and Wagner, H.P. In 'Monoclonal Antibodies and Cancer' (B. Boss, R. Langman, I.S. Trowbridge and R. Dulbecco, eds.) Academic Press, New York (1983).

THE ISOLATION AND CHARACTERIZATION OF MONOCLONAL ANTIBODIES AGAINST MURINE ALPHA FETOPROTEIN

A. I. Goussev, A. K. Yasova and O. M. Iezhneva

Laboratory of Tumor Immunochemistry and Immunodiagnosis
Cancer Research Centre
Moscow, USSR

I. INTRODUCTION

Alpha fetoprotein (AFP) is normally produced by embryonic hepatocytes and visceral endoderm of the yolk sac (1). In adult life, AFP is not produced except in hepatocarcinomas and certain teratocarcinomas. This abnormal expression of AFP in tumor-bearing individuals is of great value in diagnosis. To date, AFP has been detected by highly specific heterologous antisera which, because of batch-to-batch variations, are not standardized reagents, as would be desirable in immune diagnosis. This present communication describes the isolation and characterization of a rat anti-mouse AFP monoclonal antibody.

II. RESULTS

Hybridomas were prepared by fusion of immune August rat spleen cells with the myeloma NS-1 obtained from Dr. Milstein. Rats were immunized in the hind foot pad with 30mg of mouse AFP (AFPm), prepared by the method of Goussev et al. (2) and emulsified in complete Freund's adjuvant, and bled thirty days later to test for anti-AFPm activity. One rat (with the highest anti-AFPm titer) was boosted i.v. with 60mg AFPm in saline, and three days later the spleen was taken for fusion

using the method of Davidson and Gerald (3). Hybridoma
supernatants were assayed by enzyme—linked immunosorbent assay
(ELISA) and confirmed by indirect immunoperoxidase staining of
liver sections from rats that had been treated with carbon
tetrachloride to induce AFP synthesis. Four wells were
selected for recloning at 0.5 cell per well in 96—well trays.
Supernatants from each clone were then tested by ELISA for
binding to rat, mouse and human AFP as shown in Table 1. Of
the 47 clones assayed, 45 reacted with both rat and mouse AFP
and only two were specific for AFPm. Two clones reacted
weakly with human AFP.

TABLE 1.   Determinant Specificity of Hybridoma Anti—AFPm
            Analyzed by ELISA

F_4 Clones Selected For Recloning	No. of Wells Showing Growth of Subclones	Positive Reactions With:		
		AFPm*	AFPr*	AFPh*
C10	27	27	27	1
E2	3	3	3	0
A10	13	13	11	1/11
F9	4	4	4	0
TOTALS	47	47	45	2

*AFP of mouse, rat and human was used at 1µg/ml.

In conclusion, our hopes of obtaining a rat anti—mouse AFP
monoclonal that cross—reacted with human AFP were not fully
realized, and the antibodies which did bind human AFP were of
very low affinity. The monoclonal antibodies which are now
available will be used to study in vivo antitumor effects.

ABBREVIATIONS

AFP, alpha fetoprotein; AFPm, mouse alpha fetoprotein; ELISA, enzyme-linked immunosorbent assay.

ACKNOWLEDGMENTS

We thank Drs. G. I. Abelev and E. R. Karamova for characterizing our monoclonal antibodies by immunoisotachophoresis, and Drs. V. N. Baranov, N. V. Engelhardt, and M. N. Lazareva for immunoelectron microscopy with the monoclonal antibodies and liver sections from carbon tetrachloride-treated rats.

REFERENCES

1. Abelev, G.I. Cancer Res. 14, 295 (1971).
2. Goussev, A.I. and Yasova, A.K. Biochemistry (Russian) 35, 122, (1970).
3. Davidson, R.L. and Gerald, P.S. Methods Cell Biol. 15, 325 (1977).

USE OF ANTIBODIES TO MEMBRANE ANTIGENS IN THE STUDY OF DIFFERENTIATION AND MALIGNANCY IN THE HUMAN BREAST

Joyce Taylor-Papadimitriou, Joy Burchell
and Sidney E. Chang

Imperial Cancer Research Fund
London, United Kingdom

I. INTRODUCTION

The first attempts to develop mouse monoclonal antibodies to antigens specifically associated with carcinomas and melanomas have produced several antibodies directed against oligosaccharide determinants which may be in gangliosides or in the carbohydrate side chains of membrane or matrix glycoproteins (1-6). In parallel, antibodies to similar determinants have been produced and used as immunological markers for differentiation antigens in a variety of systems (7-11). To a large extent, the production of antibodies to similar determinants may reflect the restrictions imposed by the immune system of the mouse and by what it recognized as immunogenic. However, even with antibodies to this restricted antigenic profile, it is proving possible to gain new insights into the malignant phenotype and its relation to differentiation and to develop new approaches to the diagnosis and treatment of some of the major solid tumors. Here we will discuss the application of two monoclonal antibodies directed to the human milk fat globule (HMFG), HMFG-1 and HMFG-2[1], to the study of differentiation and malignancy in the human mammary gland and to the diagnosis of malignancy in vitro and in vivo.

---

[1]Referred to in references 9 and 10 as F1.10.F3 and F3.14.A3.

II. ANTIGENIC DETERMINANTS ON HMFG RECOGNIZED BY HMFG-1 AND HMFG-2

The oligosaccharide nature of the determinants recognized by the antibodies was suggested by a variety of observations (12) and is confirmed by the observation that binding to a delipidated preparation of HMFG, as detected in a solid-phase enzyme-linked immunosorbant assay (ELISA), is inhibited by wheat germ and peanut lectins (Figure 1). Although the oligosaccharide sequences have not yet been determined, the lectin blocking experiments predict that galactose, N-acetyl glucosamine, N-acetyl galactosamine and/or sialic acid may be included in them.

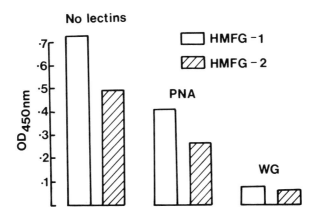

FIGURE 1. Blocking of binding of HMFG-1 and -2 to HMFG by peanut (PNA) and wheat germ (WG) lectins.

The size of the components in the HMFG which carry the determinants has been determined by staining Western blots of separated HMFG components with the antibodies in an ELISA assay. Figure 2 shows that both HMFG-1 and -2 react with high molecular weight glycoproteins (>300K). The diffuse banding

pattern is characteristic of a high carbohydrate content.
This large component of the human MFG is composed of 50%
oligosaccharide with a high proportion of galactose, N–acetyl–
glucosamine, N–acetyl galactosamine and sialic acid (13). In
reacting with oligosaccharide determinants in large molecular
weight membrane glycoproteins, HMFG–1 and –2 resemble several
other monoclonal antibodies produced using a variety of
immunogens (Table 1).

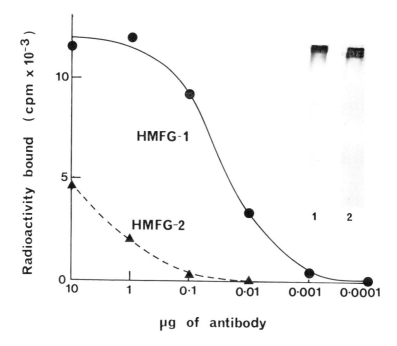

FIGURE 2. Binding of HMFG–1 and –2 to HMFG in solid–phase
radioimmunoassay and to Western blots of separated components.

III.   REACTIONS WITH SECTIONS OF BREAST TISSUE AND TUMORS

Staining of formalin–fixed paraffin–embedded sections of
lactating and resting normal gland with HMFG–1 and –2 using
the immunoperoxidase technique showed that the determinants
recognized by the antibodies were strongly expressed by the
lactating glandular epithelium but only weakly expressed in
the nonlactating breast (10).   Both antibodies, however,

TABLE 1.   Antibodies to Oligosaccharide Determinants in
Large Glycoproteins Found in Breast Carcinomas
and Other Tumors

Antibody	Immunogen	MW	Reference
HMFG-1	Delipidated HMFG	300-400K	9
HMFG-2	Delipidated HMFG and milk cells	80-400K	9
M8, M18	HMFG (not delipidated)	200-400K	11
B72.3	Membrane preparation of metastatic breast cancer	200-400K	4
Mov1	Membrane preparation from mucinous ovarian carcinoma	large mucin	14
Ca1	Hep-2 glycoproteins	350 and 390K	2
225.28S	Melanoma cells	280 and 440K	15
GICA	Colon carcinoma cells	large mucin	5

showed positive reactions with many primary and secondary
breast cancers. While the degree of reactivity varied and the
reaction of the tumor cells was not homogeneous, HMFG-2
generally gave a stronger reaction than HMFG-1 with most primary carcinomas and with all metastatic lesions from infiltrating ductal carcinomas found in lymph nodes. The antibodies therefore appear to recognize differentiation antigens
expressed on lactating breast and on breast cancers, with the
HMFG-2 determinant being more consistently conserved in the
metastatic cell.

IV. REACTIONS WITH CULTURED MAMMARY EPITHELIAL CELLS

In general, HMFG-2 reacted more positively with sections
of breast carcinoma and cell lines cultured from them, while
HMFG-1 reacted more positively (radioimmunoassay or ELISA)
with normal mammary epithelial (HumE) cells cultured from milk
(12). Kinetic studies of the association and dissociation of
purified [^{125}I]-labeled immunoglobulins using milk cells and a

breast cancer line, T47D, showed that the stronger reaction
with milk cells is due to the presence of more antigenic sites
(12).   On the other hand, the stronger binding of HMFG-2 to
T47D cells appears to be due to a higher affinity of the antibody for these cells (12).   Figure 3 shows that both antibodies bind to high affinity sites on HumE cells.   However,
the binding sites on T47D cells appear to be heterogeneous in
their affinity for the antibodies and complex dissociation
curves are seen, with HMFG-2 showing a higher proportion of
high affinity sites.   The data of Figure 3 emphasize that the
affinity of an antibody for a membrane antigen may vary
depending on the cell expressing the antigen.   This observation has practical implications for the in vivo use of antibodies for tumor localization, since it cannot be assumed that
all tumors expressing a specific antigen will exhibit similar
affinities for a particular antibody.

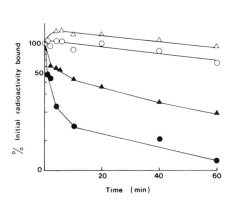

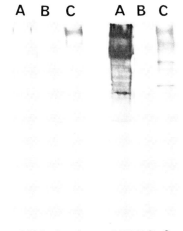

HMFG-1   HMFG-2

FIGURE 3.   Left: Dissociation of [^{125}I]-labeled HMFG-1
(●,o) and HMFG-2 (▲, Δ) from human milk epithelial (HumE)
cells (o, Δ) and T47D cells (●, ▲).   Right: Binding of the
antibodies to blots of separated components from (A) T47D, (B)
Hs578T, and (C) HumE cells.

Although both antibodies reacted with high molecular
weight components in Western blots of HMFG, a more complex

pattern of reaction is observed with blots of cell lysates (Figure 3). Whereas HMFG-1 binds with high affinity to 300–400K components of milk epithelial cells, HMFG-2 binds with high affinity to several lower molecular weight components (80–250K) in both HumE and T47D cells. The lack of binding of either antibody by any components from a nonepithelial breast cancer line, Hs578T, demonstrates the specificity of the binding. The results are consistent with the interpretation that the high affinity HMFG-1 site is present in complex carbohydrate side chains of large glycoprotein molecules while the high affinity HMFG-2 site is more abundant on simpler carbohydrate side chains of glycoproteins with a lower carbohydrate content. The difference in the antigenic sites recognized by HMFG-1 and -2 could possibly be related to the degree of branching of the oligosaccharide side chains, as is seen with the human blood group i and I antigens (7). Whether the smaller components recognized by HMFG-2 represent precursors of the larger molecules is not yet clear.

V. EXPRESSION OF HMFG-1 ANTIGEN AND REDUCED GROWTH OF NORMAL MAMMARY EPITHELIUM

Indirect immunofluorescent staining of live cultures of milk HumE cells indicates that there are many HMFG-1 sites expressed and relatively few HMFG-2 sites expressed (Figures 4A and B), confirming the data obtained from binding experiments using radiolabeled immunoglobulins (12). The material staining with the antibodies in unfixed cultures could be extracellular, as the outlines of the stained blocks do not always correspond to obvious cellular entities seen in phase pictures. In fixed cultures, the pattern of staining of HMFG-1 is similar to that seen with live cells but the level is reduced (Figure 4C). On the other hand, all the cells in fixed cultures stain with HMFG-2 and the staining is clearly cell-associated (Figure 4D). These patterns of staining suggest that the high molecular weight cellular component expressing high affinity sites for HMFG-1 may become extracellular and in live cultures form a barrier excluding large molecules like immunoglobulins. Such protection is afforded epithelial cells in vivo by surface mucins.

The production of the complex material expressing many HMFG-1 sites is associated with decreased growth of the HumE cells. HMFG-1 positive cells separated with a fluorescence-activated cell sorter (FACS) show a dramatically lower growth rate than HMFG-1 negative cells; HMFG-1 negative cells, how-

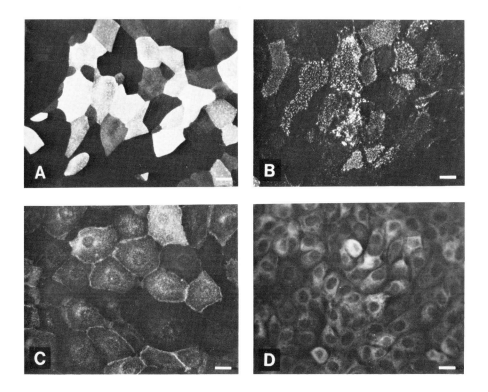

FIGURE 4.   Indirect immunofluorescent staining of live
(A,B) and methanol:acetone-fixed (C,D) milk cells with HMFG-1
(A,C) and HMFG-2 (B,D).   Bars = 20μm.

ever, can give rise to cells that express the HMFG-1 sites
(15).   These results are consistent with the idea that termin-
ally differentiated glandular mammary epithelial cells express
many antigenic determinants recognized by HMFG-1.   Although
the HMFG-2 site is more dominant in many primary carcinomas,
HMFG-1 sites are also found and their expression in this tissue may reflect the very poor growth potential of these cancer
cells in vitro.

VI. USE OF HMFG ANTIBODIES TO DETECT CANCER CELLS IN VIVO AND
    IN VITRO

The antigens recognized by the antibodies described here
are neither tumor-specific nor tissue-specific but they do
have a restricted expression, being found only on some normal
epithelial cells (those lining certain exocrine glands or
ducts) and carcinomas (10,17). HMFG-2 shows a somewhat wider
spectrum of reaction than HMFG-1, particularly in its reaction
with metastatic carcinomas, and is proving to be useful for
the identification of malignant carcinoma cells in serous
effusions (17,18). Whereas HMFG-2 shows a weak or negative
reaction with reactive mesothelial cells, it reacts positively
with mesothelioma (G. Canti, personal communication).
    The expression of these membrane antigens is almost
certainly affected by external factors, and metastatic cells
from the major types of carcinomas when found in serous effusions can express them more strongly than the original primary
carcinoma (or lymph node metastasis). Ovarian and breast
carcinoma cells in effusions have been found to be uniformly
positive with HMFG-2 and even colon carcinomas, which in the
primary site do not show a strong positive reaction, may do so
in serous effusions. This modulation by external factors in
the expression of membrane antigens, particularly those
involving oligosaccharide determinants, may complicate the use
of antibodies directed to such antigens in cancer diagnosis,
and the use of a cocktail of antibodies may be more appropriate.
    In general, the normal tissues recognized by HMFG-2 are
topographically limited to small areas lining ducts (bile,
epididymis) or to glands involved in exocrine secretion
(sweat, salivary and sebaceous glands, exocrine parts of the
pancreas, endometrium and cervix) (10). It has therefore
proved feasible to locate some carcinomas in vivo using radiolabeled antibody (19). Ovarian tumors appear to express the
HMFG-2 antigen strongly and can be detected with ^{123}I-labeled
HMFG-2 without applying a correction for nonspecific binding.
Between 0.2 and 3% of the administered radioactivity was
located in the tumor, and antibody could be detected in the
carcinoma after surgery by direct staining with peroxidase
coupled to rabbit anti-mouse immunoglobulin. Almost certainly, localization can be improved by using F(ab)$_2$ fragments
to speed up clearance of circulating antibody.
    The successful use of intact molecules of the HMFG-2
immunoglobulin can probably be attributed to three factors:
(1) the isotope ^{123}I has the right energy for detection by the

gamma scanner; (2) the antibody is of the IgG1 type, which
does not induce a host response and thus remains bound to the
antigen; (3) the nature of the antigen (oligosaccharide in a
large glycoprotein) means that many sites are present on a
single molecule with a low turnover ensuring a high and rea-
sonably stable level of binding. However, these factors are
not those required for successful immunotherapy. Such factors
would presumably include an antibody with greater specificity.
On the other hand, it may be that normal lining epithelial
cells are protected by natural barriers (basement membranes
and surface mucus) from exogeneously administered immunoglobulins, and the use of a tumor-associated rather than
tumor-specific antibody may be feasible.

VII.   COMPARISON TO OTHER ANTIBODIES RECOGNIZING SIMILAR
       ANTIGENIC DETERMINANTS

    Antibodies recognizing oligosaccharide determinants asso-
ciated with carcinomas of the intestinal tract and with melanomas have been studied in detail, and in some cases the
sequence of the sugars making up the determinant has been
elucidated (5,6,13). Many of these antibodies recognize the
lacto-fucopentaose-III sequence (6), or similar sequences
which may have a terminal sialic acid residue (5). The
$\beta D-Gal1 \rightarrow \frac{3}{4}$ glucosamine sequence contained in these
determinants may also be found in the HMFG-1 and -2
determinants, as well as in the M8 (11; C. Foster, personal
communication) and Cal determinants (2). However, these
antibodies show a spectrum of reactivity different from each
other (see Table 1) and from that shown by the antibodies
detecting antigens associated with colon carcinoma and
melanoma. Antibodies produced using tumor cells or membrane
or glycoprotein extracts (B72.3, Cal) derived from them may be
more specific for cancer cells than antibodies produced using
membrane or glycoprotein preparations from differentiated
cells (HMFG and M series). However, extensive testing of
frozen sections of normal tissues using immunological staining
techniques has not been done in all cases and until it has,
these antibodies should be regarded as tumor-associated rather
than tumor-specific.
    In experiments using lectins, changes in the patterns of
glycosylation of membrane glycoproteins have been shown to
occur both in differentiation and malignancy (20-23). In this
way, fucose and/or sialic acid have been found to be involved
in differentiation of the embryo (4,7,20,21) and skin (22) and

in the malignant transformation of colonic and mammary epithelium (23-25). By using a panel of monoclonal antibodies more
specific in their reactions than lectins, it should be possible to define more precisely these changes and to identify
glycosyl transferases which are altered in differentiating and
malignant epithelial cells.

ABBREVIATIONS

HMFG, human milk fat globule; ELISA, enzyme-linked immunosorbent assay; HumE, human mammary epithelial; FACS,
fluorescence-activated cell sorter.

REFERENCES

1. Magnani, J.L., Brockhaus, M., Smith, D.F., Ginsberg, V.,
    Blaszcyk, M., Mitchell, K.F., Steplewski, Z. and
    Koprowski, H. Science 212, 55 (1981).
2. Ashall, F., Bramwell, M.E. and Harris, H. Lancet,
    July 3, 1 (1982).
3. Pukel, C.S., Lloyd, K.O., Travassos, L.R., Dippold, W.G.,
    Oettgen, H.F. and Old, L.J. J. Exp. Med. 155, 1133
    (1982).
4. Nuti, M., Teramoto, Y.A., Mariani-Costantini, R.,
    Hand, P.H., Colcher, D. and Schlom, J. Int. J. Cancer
    29, 539 (1982).
5. Magnani, J.L., Nilsson, B., Brockhaus, M., Zop, D.,
    Steplewski, Z., Koprowski, H. and Ginsberg, V. J. Biol.
    Chem. 257, 14365 (1982).
6. Brockhaus, M., Magnani, J.L., Herlyn, M., Balszczyk, M.,
    Steplewski, Z., Koprowski, H. and Ginsberg, V. Arch.
    Biochem. Biophys. 217, 647 (1982).
7. Kapadia, A., Feizi, T. and Evans, M.J. Exp. Cell Res.
    131, 185 (1981).
8. Shevinsky, L.H., Knowles, B.B., Damjanov, I. and
    Solter, D. Cell 30, 697 (1982).
9. Taylor-Papadimitriou, J., Peterson, J.A., Arklie, J.,
    Burchell, J., Ceriani, R.L. and Bodmer, W.F. Int. J.
    Cancer 28, 17 (1981).

10. Arklie, J., Taylor-Papadimitriou, J., Bodmer, W.F., Egan, M. and Millis, R. Int. J. Cancer 28, 23 (1981).
11. Foster, C.S., Dinsdale, E.A., Edwards, P.A.W. and Neville, A.M. Virchows Arch 394, 295 (1982).
12. Burchell, J., Durbin, H. and Taylor-Papadimitriou, J. J. Immunol. (1983) in press.
13. Shimizu, M. and Yamauchi, K. J. Biochem. 91, 515 (1982).
14. Colnaghi, I.M., Canevari, S., Torre, G.D., Menard, S., Miotti, S., Regazzoni, M. and Tagliabue, E., in 'Monoclonal Antibodies and Cancer' (Proceedings of the IV Armand Hammer Cancer Symposium) (B.D. Boss, R.E. Langman, I.S. Trowbridge and R. Dulbecco, eds.), Academic Press, New York (1983).
15. Wilson, B.S., Imai, K., Natali, P.G. and Ferrone, S. Int. J. Cancer 28, 293 (1981).
16. Chang, S.E. and Taylor-Papadimitriou, J. Cell Diff. 12, 143 (1983).
17. Gatter, K.C., Abdulaziz, Z., Beverley, P., Corvalan, J.R.F., Ford, C., Lane, E.B., Mota, M., Nash, J.R.G., Pulford, K., Stein, H., Taylor-Papadimitriou, J., Woodhouse, C. and Mason, D.Y. J. Clin. Pathol. 35, 1253 (1982).
18. Epenetos, A., Canti, G., Taylor-Papadimitriou, J., Curling, M. and Bodmer, W.F. Lancet November 6, 1004 (1982).
19. Epenetos, A., Britton, K.E., Mather, S., Shepherd, J., Granowska, M., Taylor-Papadimitriou, J., Nimmon, C.C., Durbin, H., Hawkins, L.R., Malpas, J.S. and Bodmer, W.F. Lancet November 6, 999 (1982).
20. Gooi, H.C., Feizi, T., Kapadia, A., Knowles, B.B., Solter, D. and Evans, M.J. Nature 292, 156 (1981).
21. Miyauchi, T., Yonezawa, A., Takamura, T., Chiba, T., Tejima, S., Ozawa, M., Sato, E. and Muramatsu, T. Nature 299, 168 (1982).
22. Zieske, J.D. and Bernstein, I.A. J. Cell Biol. 95, 626 (1982).
23. Springer, G.F., Desai, P.R. and Banatwala, I. J. Natl. Cancer Inst. 54, 335 (1979).
24. Newman, R., Klein, P.J. and Rudland, P.S. J. Natl. Cancer Inst. 63, 1339 (1979).
25. Boland, C.R., Montgomery, C.K. and Kim, Y.S. Proc. Natl. Acad. Sci. USA 79, 2051 (1982).
26. Koprowski, H., in 'Monoclonal Antibodies and Cancer' (Proceedings of the IV Armand Hammer Cancer Symposium) (B.D. Boss, R.E. Langman, I.S. Trowbridge and R. Dulbecco, eds.). Academic Press, New York (1983).

QUESTIONS AND ANSWERS

McGEE: Using monoclonal antibodies, were you able to pick up any preinvasive lesions in breast like in duct cancer?

TAYLOR–PAPADIMITRIOU: Yes.

McGEE: How many?

TAYLOR–PAPADIMITRIOU: Everything that is not normal: some papillomas, epitheliosis, etc.

McGEE: So it not specific for preinvasive lesions?

TAYLOR–PAPADIMITRIOU: No.

DIFFERENTIAL TURNOVER RATE OF SURFACE PROTEINS IN ACTIVELY PROLIFERATING AND DIFFERENTIATED C$_6$ GLIOMA CELLS[1]

Shail K. Sharma and Rakesh Kumar

Department of Biochemistry
All India Institute of Medical Sciences
New Delhi-110029, India

U. N. Singh

Molecular Biology Unit
Tata Institute of Fundamental Research
Bombay-400005, India

I. INTRODUCTION

Brain tumor cells (neuronal and glial) in culture show distinctive morphological and physiological differentiation and offer a versatile model system for a variety of studies. The ease with which their two phases, comprising actively proliferating and morphologically differentated cells, can be experimentally manipulated has been particularly useful in such studies.

The program initiated in our group about a year ago has a two-fold objective: (i) identification and characterization of neuron-specific antigens exhibiting cellular and/or regional specificity, with particular emphasis on their onto-genetic development; and (ii) analysis of antigenic components of human brain tumors of both neuronal and glial origin. The

[1]Supported by a grant (SERC 12(1)/80-STP II) from Department of Science and Technology, Government of India.

239

approach involves use of cultured human neuroblastoma and glioma cells and cells from fetal and adult brain as heterologous antigenic stimulants in BALB/c mice. Monospecific antibodies produced by hybridomas (1) are screened for their binding to neuronal and glial cells by conventional immunohistochemical techniques. They are also examined for their cross-reactivity towards brain tumor samples obtained from surgical ablation, with a view to identifying any specific antigenic components associated with the tumorous cells.

II. C_6 GLIOMA CELLS AS A MODEL SYSTEM IN STUDIES ON DIFFERENTIATION

Generation of monoclonal antibodies against various determinants on a defined antigenic molecule is a straightforward task. The application of such antibodies, however, as a probe in studying a cellular organization comprised of unknown or ill-defined proteins demands painstaking efforts in identifying functionally meaningful species from a host of hybridoma products. Needless to say, an a priori knowledge of the nature of proteins responsible for various phenotypic expressions of cells (differentiated or tumorigenic states) would go a long way in rationalizing the procedure for selection of appropriate monoclonal antibodies.

We have been using C_6 glioma cells as a model system for delineating the antigenic components responsible for their proliferating and differentiated states. We report here some observations (based on differential turnover rates) which have tacitly suggested the involvement of a group of cell surface proteins in the transformation of actively multiplying cells into differentiated states. In these studies, C_6 glioma cells grown to submaximal confluency were labeled with ^{125}I using a lactoperoxidase-glucose oxidase method (2). After several washings with phosphate-buffered saline, the Petri dishes were divided into two groups. One group was incubated in the culture medium (DMEM + 10% fetal calf serum) and the other in the medium containing isoproterenol (0.01mM) and Ro-20 1724 (0.5mM), a potent inhibitor of cAMP phosphodiesterase (3).

FIGURE 1. Turnover rates of ^{125}I-labeled cell surface proteins separated in SDS-PAGE. Phase contrast photographs of undifferentiated and differentiated cells are shown in bottom and top panels. The inset in the middle panel indicates variations in relative amounts of radioactivity for proteins in II and III in control (C) and isoproterenol-treated (T) cells.

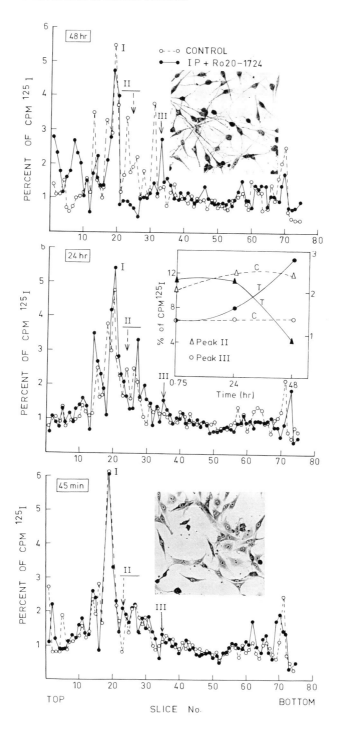

After varying periods (as shown in Figure 1), the cells were harvested. Membrane proteins were solubilized in NET buffer (NaC1, 150mM; EDTA, 5mM; Tris-HC1, 50mM, pH 7.4) containing 2% Triton X-100 and 0.1mM phenylmethyl-sulfonyl fluoride. Nuclei were removed by centrifugation at 800 x g, and the proteins in the supernatant were analyzed by sodium dodecyl sulfate-polyacrylamide gel electrophoresis (SDS-PAGE) according to the method of Laemmli (4) as modified by Ogita and Markert (5).

Figure 1 shows the labeling pattern obtained by counting 1mm thick slices of the lanes in an LKB minigamma counter. Note that the counts in different fractions were normalized and expressed as percent of total radioactivity. It is evident from the figure that a relative increase in the amount of radioactivity associated with a group of proteins (MW 65,000-80,000, marked by a bar) in the control group is almost completely abolished in the differentiated cells. This has suggested an enhanced turnover of some proteins in this group following differentiation. In contrast, a radioactive peak corresponding to a protein band with estimated size of 58,000 daltons becomes progressively more prominant after isoproterenol treatment. The contrasting behavior of the two classes of surface proteins (II and III) are shown in the inset. It is not clear at present whether this indicates differences in the turnover rates of some proteins in the two regions or whether this is due to their preferential loss or retention in the membrane matrix. In our studies with monoclonal antibodies obtained from spleen cells from mice hyperimmunized with C_6 glioma cells, we are concentrating on the proteins lying in regions II and III for a possible clue as to their role in the differentiation of these cells.

ABBREVIATIONS

SDS-PAGE, sodium dodecyl sulfate-polacrylamide gel electrophoresis.

REFERENCES

1. Kohler, G. and Milstein, C. Nature (London) 256, 495 (1975).
2. Hubbard, A.L. and Cohn, Z.A. J. Cell Biol. 64, 438 (1975).
3. Oey, J. Nature (London) 257, 317 (1975).
4. Laemmli, U.K. Nature (London) 227, 680 (1970).
5. Ogita, Z. and Markert, C.L. Anal. Biochem. 99, 233(1979).

HLA-DR EXPRESSION ON NONLYMPHOID HUMAN TUMOR CELLS: BIOCHEMICAL AND HISTOCHEMICAL STUDIES WITH MONOCLONAL ANTIBODIES[1]

G. Riethmüller, J. Johnson, R. Wank,
D. J. Schendel, H. Göttlinger and E. P. Rieber

Institute for Immunology, University of Munich
Munich, Federal Republic of Germany

J. M. Gokel

Pathology Institute, University of Munich
Munich, Federal Republic of Germany

I. INTRODUCTION

Gorer's classic discovery of histocompatibility antigens exemplifies how immunological approaches to oncology have repeatedly yielded unexpected insights for immunology itself (1). It may be relevant to the topic of this presentation to mention the early discovery by Lilly of major histocompatibility locus (MHC)-linked resistance to Gross virus leukemia, which eventually led to the definition of the immune response (or I) region in the murine MHC (2). Soon after its introduction, the hybridoma technique was applied to the search for human leukemia-associated antigens, and through this approach a number of heretofore unknown differentiation antigens were identified.

---

[1]This work was supported by Mildred Scheel Krebshilfe Foundation and Deutsche Forschungsgemeinschaft.

II. MONOCLONAL ANTIBODY 16.23 RECOGNIZES AN ALLOTYPIC DETERMINANT ON THE BETA CHAIN OF HLA-DR3

The first part of this presentation is devoted to the descrption of a monoclonal antibody which was produced by immunization with a melanoma cell line and which was found to recognize a polymorphic epitope on human Ia-like molecules. The particular monoclonal antibody was detected through the matched target pair approach, where monoclonal antibodies were screened on the immunizing melanoma cells, Epstein-Barr virus (EBV)-transformed lymphoblasts, and normal peripheral blood lymphocytes (PBL) derived from the same patient. In screening assays for binding, high reactivity to the patient's melanoma cells and B cell lines was easily detected in the absence of significant binding to PBL.

Polyacrylamide gel electrophoresis of the immunopre-cipitates revealed a typical two-chain structure with an apparent moleular weight of 37K and 31K under reducing conditions and of 34K and 26K under nonreducing conditions. For determination of the allospecificity of the monoclonal antibody, a population of DR-typed donors was tested in a microcytotoxicity test. A close association with the DR-3 alloantigen was found and occasional positivity was seen with DR-6 individuals. For confirmation, the tests were done on homozygous typing cells and showed a clear specificity for DW-3 and DW-6. Family studies indicated that the epitope recognized by the antibody 16.23 segregated with the DW-3/DR-3 haplotype (3).

Thus, antibody 16.23 was the first monoclonal antibody obtained which recognized a given allotypic specificity on human Ia-like molecules, and it could therefore be used to localize this epitope on the two-chain antigen. For this purpose, the α and β chains were separated by gel electro-phoresis and subsequently electroblotted onto nitrocellulose papers and incubated with the monoclonal antibody. After the development of the filter paper with iodinated protein A, it was shown that the antibody only bound to the separated β chain (Figure 1).

Binding inhibition of iodinated 16.23 was obtained with several, but not all, antibodies against monomorphic DR-like determinants. When expression of 16.23 epitope and mono-morphic determinants was compared in different cell popula-tions, it became evident that the 16.23 epitope was much more restricted in its expression. T lymphocytes were repeatedly negative; and, also, mitogen-stimulated lymphoblasts were labeled conspicuously less often with the 16.23 antibody

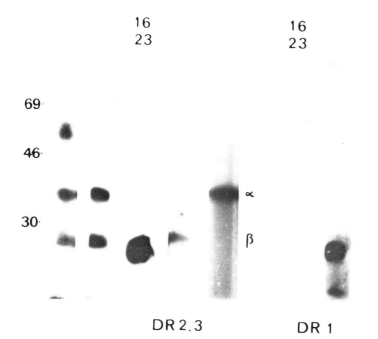

FIGURE 1.   Binding of antibody 16.23 to cell lysate
material separated by sodium dodecyl sulfate-polyacrylamide
gel electrophoresis and transferred to nitrocellulose paper.
Lanes (from left to right): 1) surface-iodinated, unboiled,
precipitated from JuSo B cell line; 2) as 1, boiled (100°C, 2
min), precipitated with 16.23; 3) unlabeled lysate, boiled,
blotted and detected with 16.23; 4) unlabeled lysate, boiled,
blotted and developed with rabbit antiserum to DR β chains;
5) same as 4, developed with antiserum to DR chains; 6) lysate
from DR1/1 B cell, unlabeled, boiled, developed with 16.23;
7) same as 6, developed with rabbit antiserum to DR β chain.
(Rabbit sera were kind gifts of Dr. J. F. Kaufman, Basel
Institute of Immunology.)

(Table 1).   In addition, no expression of the 16.23
determinant was seen on a series of alloreactive T cell clones
derived from a 16.23-positive individual, although all clones
bound monoclonal antibodies directed against monomorphic
epitopes on DR antigens. Thus, this antibody induced against
tumor cells allows a more detailed analysis of expression of
the particular epitope on different normal cells.

TABLE 1. Expression of Polymorphic and Monomorphic
HLA–DR–Associated Determinants on Nucleated
Cells from JuSo (DR 2,3) (Indirect immunofluo-
rescence).

| | Percent Positive Cells | |
	Monomorphic Moab	Moab 16,23
Melanoma cell line	100	100
EBV B cell line	100	100
PBL	20	5-6
B lymphocytes (Degalan)	73	20
T lymphocytes (E–Rosettes)	0	0
Phagocytic cells	17	0
Peroxidase$^+$ monocytes	25	24
PHA–stimulated blasts (14 d)	40	5
ConA–stimulated blasts (13 d)	42	1

Moab = monoclonal antibody

III. IN VIVO EXPRESSION OF Ia–LIKE ANTIGENS ON MAMMARY CARCINOMA CELLS AND CORRELATION WITH INFILTRATING LYMPHOCYTE SUBSETS

With the experience of finding Ia–like antigens on non–lymphoid tumor cells, we became interested in the expression of DR–like antigens on tumor cells in vivo. We have under-taken a survey on patients with primary mammary carcinomas, tumors with frequent multilocular distribution in the affected breast. Of about fifteen primary mammary carcinomas, three carcinomas were found in which a distinct expression of Ia–like antigens could be demonstrated with monoclonal antibodies against monomorphic DR–like determinants using an immuno-peroxidase staining technique.

In these patients, the most conspicuous finding was that the expression of DR antigens was distinctly heterogeneous,

i.e., tumor areas or tumor islets were either totally negative
or positive. On the same sections, we therefore identified
the infiltrating cells using monoclonal antibodies against
various T cell subpopulation-associated antigens. A striking
congruence was found in the sense that tumor areas with infiltrating cells were usually positive for expression of Ia-like
antigens, whereas Ia-negative tumor regions were not infiltrated by lymphocytes (Figure 2). The preponderant surface
antigen on the infiltrating lymphocytes was the T8 antigen (in
our nomenclature, T811), defining a 30/34K heterodimer characteristic for cytotoxic/suppressor T cells (4). In DR-
negative tumor areas, cells carrying this phenotype were found
surrounding the tumor islets in a corona-like fashion without
infiltration. In contrast to the T811$^+$ cytotoxic/suppressor
subsets infiltrating into the tumor, the T4$^+$/Leu3a$^+$ cells
(generally deemed to be helper/inducer cells) did not show a
comparable degree of infiltration but seemed to accumulate in
the outer perimeter of the tumor tissue.

These striking findings can so far be recorded only in a
descriptive manner. They demonstrate, however, how monoclonal
antibodies as molecular probes can be used to unravel the
complex local interaction of a primary tumor with the host
tissue. Whether the heterogeneity in DR expression reflects a
polyclonal state of the tumor at the time of the operation or
reflects the heterogeneity due to cell variants remains to be
determined. The biological meaning of the congruence of
infiltrating lymphocytes and tumor areas expressing DR-like
antigens is unclear at the present time. A note of caution
against premature speculations is warranted, as so often wish-
ful thinking in tumor immunology has blurred the perception of
facts. At the present time, it is difficult to establish the
actual site of DR synthesis. The role of lymphocytes cannot
be deduced merely from their surface phenotype and their
localization in the particular tumor islets. It has been
suggested by Mason and co-workers that DR expression on non-
lymphoid cells may be induced by lymphocytes when activated
during graft-versus-host or other immune reactions (5).

The clinical history of one of these patients revealed
that the tumor studied was her second mammary carcinoma within
a period of three years, the first tumor being extirpated on
the contralateral breast. This type of mammary carcinoma with
a strong inflammatory reaction is thought to be particularly
malignant. Thus, immunoselection may play a role in the
observed tumor cell diversity. It seems worthwhile to develop
an immunohistochemical examination scheme, to apply it to a
greater number of patients, and to correlate the particular
phenotype of the tumor, as well as the pattern of surrounding
lymphoid cells, with the ultimate clinical fate of the

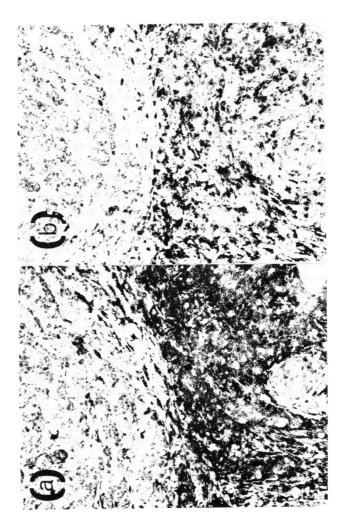

patients. Thus, one can foresee that the hybridoma technique will provide a means for dissecting the complex interactions of the heterogeneous malignant cells and cells of the immune system.

ACKNOWLEDGMENTS

We thank Renate von Carnap for help with the manuscript.

ABBREVIATIONS

MHC, main histocompatibility locus; EBV, Epstein-Barr virus; PBL, peripheral blood lymphocytes.

REFERENCES

1. Gorer, P.A. J. Pathol. Bact. 44, 691 (1937).
2. Lilly, F., Boyse, E.A. and Old, L.J. Lancet, December 5, 1207 (1964).
3. Johnson, J.P., Meo, T., Riethmüller, G., Schendel, D.J. and Wank, R. J. Exp. Med. 156, 104 (1982).
4. Rieber, E.P., Lohmeyer, J., Schendel, D.J. and Riethmüller, G. Hybridoma 1, 59 (1981).
5. Barclay, A.N. and Mason,D.W. J. Exp. Med. 156, 1665 (1982).

FIGURE 2. Immunoperoxidase Staining of Serial Sections of a Solid Mammary Carcinoma (Patient M.A.). (a) Staining with antibody directed against human Ia-like antigens (OKIa, Ortho); light upper area, DR-negative tumor region; dark lower area, DR-positive tumor cells. (b) Staining with anti-T811 (suppressor/cytotoxic subset); lower area with dispersed $T8^+$ lymphocytes.

CANCER-ASSOCIATED CARBOHYDRATE ANTIGENS DETECTED BY
MONOCLONAL ANTIBODIES

John L. Magnani and Victor Ginsburg

National Institute of Arthritis, Diabetes,
and Digestive and Kidney Diseases
National Institutes of Health
Bethesda, Maryland

I. INTRODUCTION

During differentiation and oncogenic transformation, the structures of complex carbohydrates in the cell change as a result of a modulation of the levels of glycosyltransferases. Many monoclonal antibodies which detect differentiation or transformation antigens are directed against these carbohydrates.

Cell surface carbohydrates can exist in either glycoproteins or glycolipids, and in many cases identical oligosaccharide are found on both types of molecules (1). As glycolipids have a relatively simple structure and usually contain one hapten oligosaccharide, they are ideal for the chemical characterization of cell surface carbohydrate antigens.

II. A GASTROINTESTINAL CANCER-ASSOCIATED ANTIGEN DETECTED BY MONOCLONAL ANTIBODY 19-9 IS A GANGLIOSIDE CONTAINING SIALYLATED LACTO-$\underline{N}$-FUCOPENTAOSE II IN COLORECTAL CARCINOMA CELL LINE SW 1116

The binding of two monoclonal antibodies (19-9, 52a) produced by hybridomas obtained from mice immunized with a human colon adenocarcinoma cell line is inhibited by serum

from most patients with gastrointestinal cancer, but not by
the serum of normal individuals, patients with inflammatory
bowel diseases, or most patients with other malignancies (2).
The antigen for these antibodies in the cell line used for
immunization is a monosialoganglioside (3) and was purified as
described in (4). About 30µg of ganglioside is obtained from
1 gram wet weight of tissue culture cells.

The structure of the carbohydrate was determined by methy-
lation analysis and combined gas chromatography and mass spec-
troscopy of the trifluoroacetylated derivative (4) to be:

$$NeuNAc\alpha 2-3Gal\beta 1-3GlcNAc\beta 1-3Gal\beta 1-4Glc$$
$$4$$
$$|$$
$$Fuc\alpha 1$$

This is a sialylated derivative of the normal Le^a blood
group-active pentasaccharide, lacto-N-fucopentaose II. Both
fucose and sialic acid are immunodominant sugars, as neither
lacto-N-fucopentaose II nor LS-tetrasaccharide a (the defuco-
sylated sialyloligosaccharide) binds the antibody.

Determining the structure of this carbohydrate antigen was
helpful in evaluating its genetic distribution in cancer
patients. About 5% of the population belong to the $Le^{(a-b-)}$
blood group and lack the Le gene which is responsible for the
synthesis of the $\alpha 1-4$ fucosyltransferase (5) that produces
lacto-N-fucopentaose II from lacto-N-tetraose. Tumors from
Le(a-b-) patients with gastrointestinal cancer, therefore,
cannot synthesize a sialyl derivative of lacto-N-fucopentaose
II and are negative for this antigen (6).

FIGURE 1. Distribution of Antigen Among Human Tissues.
Autoradiography of antigens on thin-layer chromatograms was
performed as described in (4). Antibody 19-9 was used. The
amount of extract chromatographed expressed as the volume of
packed cells from which it was obtained is as follows: lane
1, 2µl normal intestinal mucosa; lane 2, 2µl of primary colon
adenocarcinoma; lane 3, 0.5µl of liver metatasis of pancreatic
carcinoma; lane 4, 1µl of colorectal carcinoma cell line
SW 1116; lane 5, 1µl of meconium; lane 6, 1µl of melanoma cell
line WM 9; lane 7, 1µl of brain gangliosides; lane 8, 1µg of
normal spleen; and lane 9, 1µl of erythrocytes. The positions
of some standard gangliosides and neutral glycolipids are
shown on the left.

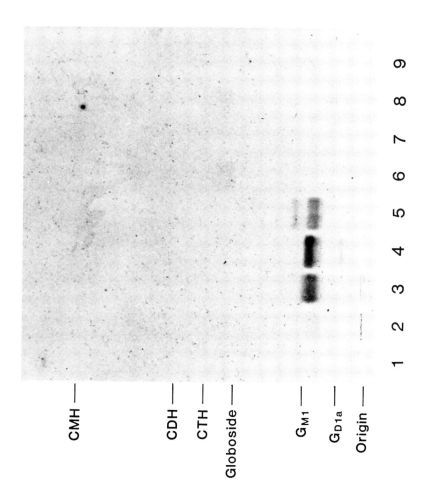

The distribution of the carbohydrate antigen among human tissues was analyzed by autoradiography of thin-layer chromatograms staining with monoclonal antibody followed by ^{125}I-labeled goat anti-mouse IgG (3,4). As shown in Figure 1, antigen with the same mobility as the monosialoganglioside (lane 4) was detected in extracts of two carcinomas (lanes 2 and 3) and in extracts of meconium (lane 5). The small amount of antigen with a lower mobility detected in the extract of the colon carcinoma cell line is probably an octasaccharide by analogy to other glycolipids:

NeuNAcα2-3Galβ1-3GlcNAcβ1-3Galβ1-3GlcNAcβ-3Galβ1-4Glc
                                                  4
                                                  |
                          Fucα1

Antigen, possibly glycoprotein, was detected at the origin of both carcinoma extracts. No antigen was detected in extracts of normal intestinal mucosa, normal spleen, erythrocytes, a melanoma cell line, or in human brain gangliosides. By immunoperoxide staining of normal tissue sections, however, antigen was detected in a layer of ductal cells in normal pancreas and a layer of secretory cells in the normal salivary glands and bronchial epithelium (7).

III.   SIALYLATED LACTO-N-FUCOPENTAOSE II IS PRESENT ON A MUCIN
        IN PATIENT'S SERA

Although the human adenocarcinoma cell line used for immunization of mice contained a ganglioside antigen, based on the following criteria the antigen in serum of cancer patients is a mucin.

A.   Under conditions of thin-layer chromatography where the monosialoganglioside antigen migrates halfway up the plate, the serum antigen remains at the origin as detected by radioactive antibodies and autoradiography.

B.   Upon gel filtration of serum on Sephacryl S-400, antigen is eluted in the void volume indicating an $M_r \gtrless 5 \times 10^6$. The same profile is obtained if serum is chromatographed with or without 4M Guanidine HCl, eliminating the possibility of existence of immune complexes.

C.   Incubation for 5 hours at 37°C in 0.1 N NaOH destroys the serum antigen but does not affect the ganglioside antigen.

D.   The density of the serum antigen as determined in a CsCl gradient is 1.50g/ml; in 4M guanidine-HCl in CsCl its density is 1.43g/ml.

E. The serum antigen of a cancer patient with an Le(a–b+) blood type, affinity purified by antibody 19–9, also binds anti–Le[b] monoclonal antibodies, consistent with the multiple antigenic specificities exhibited by mucins.

IV. MONOCLONAL ANTIBODIES DIRECTED AGAINST THE HUMAN Le[b] BLOOD
    GROUP

Four monoclonal antibodies produced by hybridomas obtained from a mouse immunized with the same human adenocarcinoma cell line SW 1116 (8) are directed against the Le[b] antigen of the human Lewis blood group system. Three of the antibodies (1116NS10, 1116NS33a and 1116NS38a) are of the IgM type while antibody 1116NS43a is of the IgG1 type. Their specificities were established by binding studies using purified Le[b]–active ceramide hexasaccharide and by hapten inhibition studies using purified oligosaccharides obtained from human milk (9).
The Le[b] antigen contains the terminal sugar sequence

$$Fuc\alpha1-2Gal\beta1-3GlcNAc\beta1-3Gal$$
$$4$$
$$|$$
$$Fuc\alpha1$$

and occurs in the glycolipids and glycoproteins of approximately 75% of the population who belong to the Le(a–b+ blood group. The apparent specificity of the antibodies for colorectal carcinoma cell lines (8) may be explained by the high levels of Le[a]– and Le[b]–active glycolipids that occur in some adenocarcinomas of colon and pancreas (10).

V. MANY MONOCLONAL ANTIBODIES WITH APPARENT SPECIFICITY TO
    HUMAN TUMORS ARE DIRECTED AGAINST LACTO–N̲–FUCOPENTAOSE III

Another carbohydrate antigen which occurs on both glycoproteins and glycolipids is remarkably immunogenic to the mouse. This oligosaccharide, first isolated from normal human milk and characterized in 1969 by Kobata and Ginsburg (11) is lacto–N̲–fucopentaose III.

$$Gal\beta1-4GlcNAc\beta1-3Gal\beta1-4Glc$$
$$3$$
$$|$$
$$Fuc\alpha1$$

Glycolipids containing this structure known as
Le^x or x hapten accumulate in adenocarcinomas of the
colon (12). Recently, many laboratories have produced monoclonal antibodies to human tissues for different reasons and
have found that all bind to lacto-N-fucopentaose III. Table 1
lists only those antibodies that have been published. We have
received over 200 monoclonal antibodies from different
laboratories, and approximately 20-30% of the antibodies are
directed against lacto-N-fucopentaose III.

TABLE 1.   Monoclonal Antibodies That Bind Lacto-N-
           Fucopentaose III

Monoclonal Antibody	Immunogen	Target	Reference
MY-1	promyelocytic cell line HL-60	HL-60 cells	Huang et al. (1983) Blood 61, 1020
SSEA-1	murine teratocarcinoma cell line F-9	F-9 cells	Hakomori et al. (1981) Biochem. Biophys. Res. Commun. 100, 1578
WGHS 29.1	primary gastric adenocarcinoma	colorectal cancer cells	Brockhaus et al. (1982) Arch. Bioch. Biophys. 217, 647
ZWG 13 ZWG 14 ZWG 111	liver metastasis of colon adeno-carcinoma	colorectal cancer cells	Brockhaus et al. (1982) Arch. Bioch. Biophys. 217, 647
534F8 538F12 + 19 others	small lung cell cancer line NCI-H69	lung cancer cells	Huang et al.. (1983) Arch. Bioch. Biophys. 220, 318

Specificity was determined by autoradiography of thin-layer chromatograms of glycolipids, by solid-phase radio-immunoassays and by hapten inhibition studies. Interestingly, all of these antibodies are of the IgM isotype.

In the mouse, lacto-N-fucopentaose III has been identified as the stage-specific embryonic antigen, SSEA-1 (13,14). It has been found on murine embryonal carcinoma cell line F-9 and is transiently expressed on murine embryos from the 8-cell stage up to the morula stage.

Although lacto-N-fucopentaose III is a well known component of normal human milk, antibodies to this oligosaccharide may be useful when restricted to certain cell types. The anti-MY-1 antibody produced by hybridomas obtained from a mouse immunized with HL-60 human promyelocytic leukemia cells binds significantly to granulocytes and granulocytic precursor cells but not with normal peripheral blood lymphocytes, monocytes, platelets or red cells. Furthermore, the antigen is developmentally regulated, appearing first at the promyelocytic cell stage and continuing up to mature granulocytes (15).

VI. SUMMARY

Three carbohydrate specificities of monoclonal antibodies produced against human tumors are described. The first, which is associated with gastrointestinal cancer, contains the antigenic sequence in sialylated lacto-N-fucopentaose II

$$\text{NeuNAc}\alpha 2\text{-}3\text{Gal}\beta 1\text{-}3\text{GlcNAc}\beta 1\text{-}3\text{Gal}$$
$$4$$
$$|$$
$$\text{Fuc}\alpha 1$$

In the tumor cell line used for immunization, the sequence is found on both hexasaccharide and octasaccharide ceramides. The antigen in the serum of cancer patients is attached to a mucin molecule through an O-glycosyl linkage of GalNAc to either serine or threonine.

The second carbohydrate antigen is the normal Le^b-active oligosaccharide found on both glycolipids and glycoproteins.

$$Fuc\alpha1\text{-}2Gal\beta1\text{-}3GlcNAc\beta1\text{-}3Gal$$
$$4$$
$$|$$
$$Fuc\alpha1$$

The level of this antigen is elevated in colorectal and pancreatic tumors of both Le(a+b-) and Le(a-b+) individuals (10). Monoclonal anti-Le[b] antibodies should also be useful as specific high quality reagents for routine blood analysis.

The last antigen, which is extremely immunogenic in the mouse, contains the antigenic sequence in lacto-N-fucopentaose III.

$$Gal\beta1\text{-}4GlcNAc\beta1\text{-}3Gal$$
$$3$$
$$|$$
$$Fuc\alpha1$$

This antigen is present in larger oligosaccharides in both glycoproteins and glycolipids. Although this oligosaccharide is found in normal human tissues, when restricted to hematopoietic cells it is a differentiation marker of the myeloid cells.

ACKNOWLEDGMENTS

Much of this work was performed with colleagues who have recently left this laboratory. They are Dr. Laura C. Huang (present location: University of Virginia School of Medicine, Charlottesville, VA) and Dr. M. Brockhaus (present location: Basel Institute for Immunology, Basel, Switzerland). We would also like to thank Julie Maltagliati for typing the manuscript and David B. Magnani for his meconium.

REFERENCES

1. Rauvala, H. and Finne, J. FEBS Letters 97, 1 (1979).
2. Koprowski, H., Herlyn, M. and Steplewski, A. Science 212, 53 (1981).
3. Magnani, J.L., Brockhaus, M., Smith, D.F., Ginsburg, V., Blaszczyk, M., Mitchell, K.F., Steplewski, A. and Koprowski, H. Science 212, 55 (1981).
4. Magnani, J.L., Nilsson, B., Brockhaus, M. Zopf, D., Steplewski, Z., Koprowski, H. and Ginsburg, V. J. Biol. Chem. 257, 14365 (1982).
5. Grollman, E.F., Kobata, A. and Ginsburg, V. J. Clin. Invest. 48, 1489 (1969).
6. Koprowski, H., Blaszczyk, M., Steplewski, Z., Brockhaus, M., Magnani, J.L. and Ginsburg, V. Lancet, June 12, 1332 (1982).
7. Atkinson, B.F., Ernst, C.S., Herlyn, M., Steplewski, Z., Sears, H.F. and Koprowski, H. Cancer Res. 42, 4820 (1982).
8. Koprowski, H., Steplewski, Z., Mitchell, K., Herlyn, M., Herlyn, D. and Fuhrer, P. Somatic Cell Genet. 5, 957 (1979).
9. Brockhaus, M., Magnani, J.L., Blaszcyzk, M., Steplewski, Z., Koprowski, H., Karlsson, K-A., Larson, G. and Ginsburg, V. J. Biol. Chem. 256, 1322 (1981).
10. Hakomori, S. and Andrews, H.D. Biochim. Biophys. Acta 202, 225 (1970).
11. Kobata, A. and Ginsburg, V. J. Biol. Chem. 244, 5496 (1969).
12. Yang, H-J. and Hakomori, S. J. Biol. Chem. 246, 1192 (1971).
13. Hakomori, S., Nudelman, E., Levery, S., Solter, D. and Knowles, B.B. Biochem. Biophys. Res. Commun. 100, 1578 (1981).
14. Gooi, H.C., Feizi, T., Kapadla, A., Knowles, B.B., Solter, D., Evans, M.J. Nature 292, 156 (1981).
15. Civin, C.I., Mirro, J. and Banquerigo, M.L. Blood 57, 842 (1981).

QUESTIONS AND ANSWERS

BERNSTEIN: Is there a difference between anti-Le^x antibodies in the way they recognize the carbohydrate; is there a difference in their spectrum of reactivity with different cells?

MAGNANI: Some antibodies directed against lacto-N-fucopentaose III ceramide preferentially bind glycolipids with longer saccharide chains.   These antibodies are described in Arch. Biochem. Biophys. 217, 647-651 (1982).   As illustrated in Figure 4 of that reference, antibody WGH5 29-1 will bind to lacto-N-fucopentaose III ceramide relative to the higher molecular weight glycolipids better than antibodies ZWG13, ZWG14, or ZWG111.

We have not looked for a difference in their spectrum of reactivity with different cells.

TAYLOR-PAPADIMITRIOU: Is the sialylated Le^a antigen expressed only in glycoprotein and not in glycolipids on colon tumors?

Comment: The production of monoclonal antibodies reacting with very similar groups (lacto-fucopentaose III, II, etc.) focuses on the problem of the limitation on antibody specificity imposed by the immune system of the mouse.   Will this restriction be too limiting and preclude the development of more antibodies with an absolute specificity for human tumors?

MAGNANI: In two colon tumors that we have extracted, most (but not all) of the antigen was present in glycoproteins.

MAPPING OF ANTIGENIC SITES ON HUMAN TRANSFERRIN
BY MONOCLONAL ANTIBODIES

V. Viklický, J. Bártek, H. Verlová, P. Dráber, V. Hořejší

Czechoslovak Academy of Sciences
Institute of Molecular Genetics
Prague, Czechoslovakia

I. INTRODUCTION

Transferrin is a plasma transport protein which has become a subject of interest not only for hematologists but also for oncologists, cell biologists and specialists in cell cultivation. Transferrin levels in the blood vary in a variety of pathological states, including some tumors cases. Membrane receptors for transferrin (TF) are expressed on tumor cells and growth-stimulated cells and are considered to be a characteristic of proliferating cells. We have decided to prepare a panel of monoclonal antibodies against human transferrin in order to study in detail the role of transferrin and its interaction with its specific cell membrane receptor.

II. RESULTS

Hybridomas were prepared by fusion of spleen cells from BALB/c mice immunized against human transferrin with myeloma cells X63 Ag8.653. After repeated cloning, a panel of nine monoclonal antibodies was obtained; all nine monoclonal antibodies were found to belong to the IgG1 subclass (kappa light chain), and to react only with transferrin in a mixture of plasma proteins. As most of the routinely used diagnostic tests for quantitative follow-up of transferrin are based on precipitation by antibodies, our monoclonal antibodies were

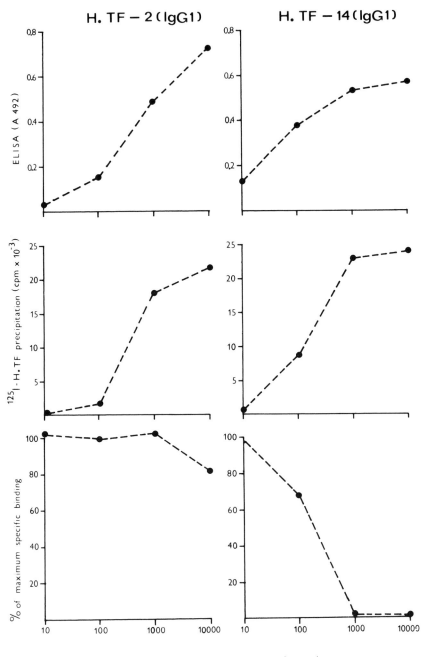

Antibody concentration (ng/ml)

FIGURE 1

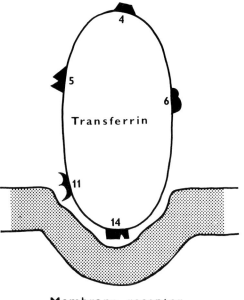

Membrane receptor

FIGURE 2

tested for their ability to precipitate the antigen. No precipitation was observed with single antibodies or with pairs;
however, several different precipitating triads have been
found. These results suggest that the monoclonal antibodies
which form precipitates when mixed bind to different antigenic
determinants of the transferrin molecule. Each monoclonal
antibody binds to intact as well as ^{125}I-labeled transferrin,
as shown by results of enzyme immunoassay and polyethylene
glycol-induced precipitation of immune complexes formed by
single monoclonal antibodies and isotope-labeled transferrin
in solution.

The ability to inhibit the interaction of transferrin with
the TF receptors of human lymphoblastoid cell line MOLT-3
differs markedly when different monoclonal antibodies are
preincubated with ^{125}I-labeled TF. Figure 1 shows the type of
results obtained with a noninhibiting antibody (HTF-2) and an
inhibiting one (HTF-14). The monoclonal antibody HTF-11 is
partially inhibiting, while all remaining antibodies in our
panel have very little, if any, effect on transferrin-
transferrin receptor interaction.

The ability of our monoclonal antibodies to bind to cell
membrane receptor-bound transferrin was also investigated. In
indirect immunofluorescence, monoclonal antibodies HTF-4, -5,

-6 and -2 could be used for detection of TF-receptor, while the receptor-bound transferrin was not detected using monoclonal antibody HTF-11 and -4.

The combined results from these precipitation tests, immunofluorescence studies and blocking tests give us some idea about the determinants on the transferrin molecule with which the individual monoclonal antibodies react. Loss of observable HTF-14 binding on the TF-receptor complex and effective blocking of TF to its receptor suggest that, for HTF-14, the target antigenic determinant is buried in, or adjacent to, transferrin's receptor binding site (Figure 2). By similar reasoning, monoclonal antibody HTF-11 is seen to react with a determinant located a short distance from the cell receptor binding site. The observations that HTF-2, -4, -5, and -6 bind to TF-receptor complexes and that they do not inhibit TF binding to its receptor suggest that the portion of the TF molecule carrying the target determinants for these monoclonal antibodies is quite distant from the receptor binding site. These results show that our panel of monoclonal antibodies can be used in mapping the antigenic determinants of transferrin and in determining its orientation after binding to the receptor. Together with monoclonal antibodies against TF-receptor, they represent useful tools in studying the biological function of transferrin.

ABBREVIATIONS

TF, transferrin.

APPLICATION OF TUMOR-LOCALIZING 791T/36 MONOCLONAL ANTIBODY IN RADIOIMMUNODETECTION OF EXPERIMENTAL AND HUMAN TUMORS AND TARGETING CYTOTOXIC DRUGS SUCH AS VINDESINE AND METHOTREXATE[1]

R. W. Baldwin, M. J. Embleton and M. V. Pimm

Cancer Research Campaign Laboratories
University of Nottingham
Nottingham, United Kingdom

I. INTRODUCTION

Developments in hybridoma technology leading to the production of monoclonal antibodies recognizing tumor-associated antigens are providing new approaches for the radioimmunodetection of tumors by external imaging of radio-nuclide-labeled antibodies (1-3). Tumor-localizing monoclonal antibodies also have considerable potential for targeting therapeutic agents in that they provide a means for the selective delivery of drugs to a local tumor, or more parti-cularly to metastases (4). These developments are illustrated in a series of studies in which a monoclonal antibody (79IT/36) initially raised against a human osteogenic sarcoma (5) has been used for the radioimmunodetection of tumors (1,6) and for developing conjugates with cytotoxic drugs (7,8) and immunomodulating agents (9).

---

[1]These studies were supported by grants from the Cancer Research Campaign.

II. IN VIVO LOCALIZATION OF RADIOISOTOPE-LABELED ANTITUMOR MONOCLONAL ANTIBODY IN HUMAN TUMOR XENOGRAFTS

Fundamental to all of the approaches proposed for targeting agents attached to monoclonal antibodies is the requirement to show that antibody preparations do localize specifically in tumors following injection into tumor-bearing hosts. This is exemplified by studies on the organ distribution of ^{131}I-labeled anti-osteogenic sarcoma monoclonal antibody (^{131}I-791T/36) in human tumor xenografts developing in CBA mice immunodeprived by thymectomy, whole body irradiation and cytosine arabinoside treatment (6). Following injection of ^{131}I-labeled antibody, there was preferential localization of radioactivity in 791T osteogenic sarcoma xenografts as assessed by the tissue:blood ratios of tumor tissue and normal organs. This localization was not due simply to abnormal blood distribution in the tumor, since simultaneously injected normal mouse IgG2b (labeled with ^{125}I) did not localize in tumors (6). The simultaneous injection of ^{131}I-791T/36 antibody and ^{125}I-normal IgG2b into tumor-bearing mice also allows one to calculate the degree of specific to nonspecific binding of immunoglobulins to tumors. This can be expressed as a localization index:

$$\frac{\text{tissue:blood ratio } ^{131}I\text{-labeled antibody}}{\text{tissue:blood ratio } ^{125}I\text{-labeled normal IgG}}$$

On this basis, the localization index for 791T/36 antibody in osteogenic sarcoma 791T was 6:1 compared to a value of 1:1 in liver (6).

Organ distribution studies with radioisotope-labeled 791T/36 antibody were further extended, since for targeting therapeutic agents it is necessary to define more precisely factors which influence tumor localization. This includes the relationship between tumor size and the extent of antibody localization, as well as the influence of antibody dose on tumor uptake. In relation to tumor size, it was established that there was a direct proportionality between the mass of subcutaneous 791T xenografts and the amount of antibody localized within the tumor (6). This is illustrated by the data in Figure 1, in which the uptake of ^{125}I-labeled 791T/36 antibody was determined two days after injection into mice bearing osteogenic sarcoma 791T xenografts ranging in size from 50mg to 820mg. There is a statistically significant correlation ($r^2 = 0.85$, p<0.01) between tumor mass and the proportion of the total body count of ^{131}I in the tumor. From the slope of the regression line, it was calculated that at the time of analysis (two days), tumors contained (0.034%) of the surviving body radioactivity/mg tissue. It was further established that with doses up to 100µg there was a direct proportionality between the amount of antibody injected intraperitoneally and its localization in 791T tumor xenografts. Above this dose, the proportion of antibody localizing in tumor decreased, with 1 to 2mg antibody being sufficient to 'saturate' tumors (mean 300mg). Since antibody uptake is directly proportional to tumor mass (Figure 1), it is feasible to extrapolate from these two sets of data and predict the dose of antibody which would effectively saturate tumors. For example, taking a saturating dose to be 1mg of 791T/36 antibody for a 300mg tumor, a tumor of 10mg would be saturated following administration of 30µg antibody. These studies also established that 0.34% of the body burden of antibody would be localized in such a 10mg tumor two to three days after injection of ^{125}I-791T/36 antibody. Taking the body burden of radiolabeled antibody at this time as 22% of the injected dose (10), this indicates that there would be on the order of 20ng antibody localized in the tumor. One of the major variables in these studies was the rate of elimination of antibody from individual mice, including both tumor-bearing ones and controls (6,10). For example, in one experiment the body burden, three days following injection of a single preparation of ^{125}I-labeled 791T/36 antibody in CBA mice, ranged between 6.3% and 26% of the injected dose (10). This variability must be taken into consideration with respect to antibody targeting of antitumor agents.

III. TUMOR DETECTION BY EXTERNAL IMAGING OF RADIONUCLIDE-LABELED 791T/36 ANTIBODY

Experimental studies with immunodeprived mice bearing xenografts of osteogenic sarcoma 791T showed that tumors could be detected by external gamma camera imaging following injection of 0.7 - 3MBq of ^{131}I or ^{123}I-labeled 791T/36 antibody (6). Imaging was carried out one to three days after antibody injection. Before imaging, mice received an i.v. injection of ^{99m}Tc pertechnetate to facilitate compensation for radiolabeled antibody in blood and extravascular spaces.

Following the imaging of ^{131}I-791T/36 antibody in human tumor xenografts, a trial was initiated to examine the potential of this antibody for detecting human tumors. This approach was considered feasible since detailed studies of the antibody established that it reacted not only with osteogenic sarcomas, but also with cells from other more common tumors including colon carcinoma. In the first trial (1), patients with primary and/or metastatic colorectal tumors received 200µg 791T/36 antibody labeled with 70 MBq ^{131}I. Imaging of the patients was carried out one, two or three days after antibody infusion with computerized image enhancement following blood labeling with ^{99m}Tc pertechnetate or ^{113m}In indium chloride.

Eleven patients with primary or metastatic tumors were reported in the first trial (1), and in nine of them accurate localization was reported (Table 1). In one patient, localization was masked because of the disposition of the tumor in relation to the urinary bladder (which gave an image due to excreted ^{131}I). Antibody did not localize in another tumor in a patient receiving local radiotherapy (30Gy). However, it was notable that in one patient a brain metastasis was identified and the antibody localized in liver metastases. Also, as shown in Table 1, the tumor:nontumor ratio of uptake of radioactivity was up to 8:1. Although only a limited number of patients have been evaluated, these findings do suggest that antibody conjugates should localize preferentially in tumors.

IV. DRUG TARGETING STUDIES

Monoclonal antibodies are being evaluated for targeting to tumors various types of therapeutic agents including bacterial/plant toxins, cytotoxic drugs, immunomodulating agents and radioactive isotopes (11). Of these approaches, we have initially elected to evaluate antibodies for targeting antitumor agents including adriamycin (12), vindesine (7) and methotrexate (8). Interferon-antibody conjugates also have been examined as a means of generating activation of natural killer cells in the environment of tumor cells (9).

A. Vindesine Conjugates

The development of antibody conjugates for targeting cytotoxic drugs is illustrated by a recent series of investigations using vindesine linked to anti-osteogenic sarcoma 791T/36 antibody. These conjugates, prepared from desacetyl-vinblastine acid hydrazide by a modification of the procedure described by Conrad and co-workers (1979), retain most of the original antibody activity and contain six moles drug per mole antibody (7,13).

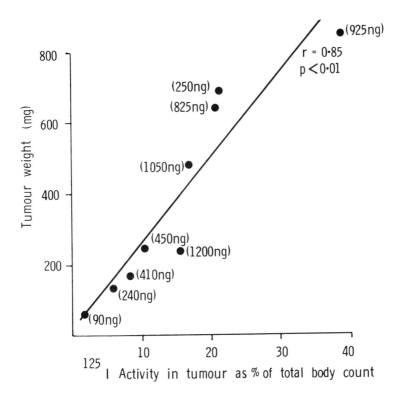

FIGURE 1. Correlation between mass of osteogenic sarcoma 791T xenografts and the tumor uptake of ^{125}I-labeled 791T/36 antibody. Tumor-bearing mice receiving [125]I-791T/36 antibody intraperitoneally were killed after two days and organ distribution of radioactivity determined. The radioactivity in tumor is expressed as a percentage of the total body radioactivity. The figures in parentheses indicate the absolute amount of antibody radioactivity within tumors.

Vindesine-791T/36 conjugates were tested for cytotoxicity against various tumor cell lines in comparison with free vindesine (VDS) after confirming by competitive binding experiments that the conjugates retained antibody activity. The conjugate and the parent drug were assayed for their ability to inhibit the uptake of ^{75}Se-selenomethionine by the target cells, it having been established that ^{75}Se-uptake correlated

TABLE 1.   External Imaging Of Colorectal Carcinomas With
[131]I-Labeled 791T/36 Monoclonal Antibody

Patient Number	Macroscopic Tumor	Site of Image	Tumor to Nontumor Ratio*
1	Primary carcinoma	Primary in pelvis	8.0:1
2	Primary carcinoma	Primary in pelvis	2.1:1
3	Primary carcinoma	Negative (behind bladder)	
4	2 primary carcinomas	Both primaries	2.1:1
5	Primary carcinoma	Primary in pelvis	1.5:1
6	Disseminated carcinoma, omental metastasis	Primary pelvis mass and secondary	
7	Disseminated carcinoma, liver metastasis	Liver metastasis	5.1:1
8	Disseminated carcinoma, liver metastasis	Liver metastasis	4.4:1
9	Inoperable carcinoma, treated by radiol therapy (30Gy)	Negative	
10	Disseminated carcinoma, liver and brain metastases	Liver and brain metastases	4.0:1
11	Disseminated carcinoma, pelvic recurrence	Recurrent tumor	4.3:1

* Tumor to nontumor ratio is the ratio of radioactivity con-
centrated over the area of the macroscopic tumor, divided by
the mean radioactivity in adjacent areas.

extremely well with the numbers of surviving cells. Repre-
sentative results of the cytotoxicity of 791T/36 antibody
conjugates on various target cells are summarized in Table 2.
In these experiments target cells were treated for 15 minutes
with VDS-antibody conjugates, then washed and cultured for 24
hours.   Cells were then labeled for 16 hours with ^{75}Se-
selenomethionine. Treatment with conjugate markedly inhibited
osteogenic sarcoma cells which bind the antibody (791T, 788T,
2 OS, T278), but conjugates had no effect upon other targets
such as ovarian carcinoma (PA1), malignant melanoma (RPMI
5966, Mel-57) and bladder carcinoma (T24) which do not express

the 791T/36 antibody-defined antigen. This was not due to any
inherent resistance to VDS, since in control studies all the
cell lines tested were susceptible to VDS-induced cytotoxicity
(7). Also, it should be noted that 791T/36 antibody alone was
not cytotoxic for antibody-binding cells (791T, 788T, 2 OS,
T278), although antibody binding can initiate complement-
mediated lysis (16).

TABLE 2.   Inhibition of Cell Survival Following Treatment
           With 791T/36-Vindesine Conjugate

| Cell Line | Antibody Binding* | % Inhibition of ^{75}Se-Methionine Uptake at Following Concentration** | | |
		40µg/ml	20µg/ml	10µg/ml
791T	++	75	73	58
788T	++	59	36	42
2 OS	+	77	78	90
T278	+	65	60	58
RPMI 5966	−	2	2	3
Mel-57	−	5	10	2
PA-1	−	3	4	1
T24	−	4	−14	0

*   Determined by radioimmunoassay and flow cytometry (5,7).
** Concentration expressed as µg/ml vindesine. The % inhibi-
    tion of ^{75}Se-methionine is expressed relative to that in
    controls treated with phosphate-buffered saline (7).

B.   Methotrexate Conjugates

    Conjugates of 791T/36 antibody with methotrexate have also
been synthesized (8). In this case, methotrexate (MTX) was
initially coupled to human serum albumin (HSA) as a carrier
and the MTX-HSA product linked to antibody. The use of HSA as
a carrier molecule allowed the attachment of larger amounts of
MTX to antibody, products containing up to 32 MTX
residues/antibody molecule being prepared.   MTX-antibody
conjugates together with free drug and HSA-MTX conjugates were
also assayed for tumor cell cytotoxicity by inhibition of
tumor cell uptake of ^{75}Se-selenomethionine.   As shown in
Table 3, treatment of target cells expressing the 791T/36

antibody-defined antigen (osteogenic sarcomas 791T and T278) with MTX-791T/36 antibody conjugates produced a cytotoxic response, whereas target cells not binding the antibody (bladder carcinoma T24, melanoma 5966) were not affected.

TABLE 3. Inhibition of Cell Survival Following Treatment With 791T/36-Human Serum Albumin-Methotrexate Conjugate

Cell Line	Antibody Binding*	% Inhibition of ^{75}Se-methionine Uptake at Following Concentrations**		
		40μg/ml	20μg/ml	10μg/ml
791T	++	79	82	79
T278	+	73	79	81
T24	–	7	0	0
RPMI 5966	–	-5	29	9

* Determined by radioimmunoassay and flow cytometry (5,7).
** Concentration expressed as μg/ml methotrexate. The % inhibition of ^{75}Se-methionine uptake is relative to that in controls treated with phosphate-buffered saline (7).

V. CONCLUSIONS

Radioimmunodetection of primary and metastatic colorectal carcinomas has been achieved by external imaging following injection of radiolabeled 791T/36 antibody (1). These investigations establish the potential of this approach for tumor detection, but in addition establish that adequate discrimination between tumor and nontumor tissues can be achieved suggesting that tumor-localizing antibody can be used for targeting antitumor agents. Developing from these studies, it has been established that 791T/36 antibody can be linked to antitumor agents including cytotoxic drugs and immuno-modulating agents (interferon) so as to retain both antibody- and drug-related activities. The therapeutic potential in vivo of these antibody conjugates has not yet been adequately evaluated, although preliminary studies indicate that VDS-791T/36 suppresses growth of osteogenic sarcoma 791T at doses which are nontoxic (15). Also, adriamycin linked via a dextran bridge to a monoclonal antibody reacting with a rat mammary carcinoma Sp4 (Adria-Sp4/A4) was more effective than free adriamycin or adriamycin linked to normal rat IgG in suppressing subcutaneous tumor growth (12). Added to this, it has been established that 791T/36 antibody conjugates with vindesine or interferon do localize in osteogenic sarcoma xenografts (Pimm, to be published), and the related investigations on the kinetics of radiolabeled antibody uptake into tumors (4,6,10) allow the design of protocols to maximize localization of antibody conjugates in tumors.

ABBREVIATIONS

VDS, vindesine; MTX, methotrexate; HSA, human serum albumin.

ACKNOWLEDGMENTS

Vindesine conjugates were prepared by Dr. G. Rowland, Lilly Research Centre, Surrey, UK. We thank our colleague, Dr. M. Garnett, for permission to present the methotrexate studies.

REFERENCES

1. Farrands, P.A., Perkins, A.C., Pimm, M.V., Hardy, J.G., Embleton, M.J., Baldwin, R.W. and Hardcastle, J.D. Lancet 397 (1982).
2. Berche, C., Mach, J-P., Lumbroso, H-D., Langlais, C., Aubry, F., Buchegger, F., Carrel, S., Rougier, P., Parmentier, C. and Tubiana, M. Br. Med. J. 285, 1447 (1982).
3. Epenetos, A.A., Mather, S., Granowska, M., Nimmon, C.C., Hawkins, L.R., Britton, K.E., Shepherd, J., Taylor-Papadimitriou, J., Durbin, H., Malpas, J.S. and Bodmer, W.F. Lancet 999 (1982).
4. Baldwin, R.W. and Pimm, M.V. Cancer Metastasis Rev. 2 ,89 (1983).
5. Embleton, M.J., Gunn, B., Byers, V.S. and Baldwin, R.W. Br. J. Cancer 43, 582 (1981).

6. Pimm, M.V., Embleton, M.J., Perkins, A.C., Price, M.R.,
    Robins, R.A., Robinson, G.R. and Baldwin, R.W.   Int. J.
    Cancer 30, 75 (1982).
7. Embleton, M.J., Rowland, G.F., Simmonds, R.G.,
    Jacobs, E., Marsden, C.H. and Baldwin, R.W.   Br. J.
    Cancer 47, 43 (1983).
8. Garnett, M., Embleton, M.J., Jacobs, E. and Baldwin, R.W.
    Int. J. Cancer 31, 661 (1983).
9. Baldwin, R.W., Flannery, G.R., Pelham, J.M. and Gray,
    J.D. Proc. Amer. Assn. Cancer Res. 23, 254 (1982).
10. Pimm, M.V. and Baldwin, R.W. In preparation (1983).
11. Baldwin, R.W., Embleton, M.J. and Price, M.R. Molec.
    Aspects Med. 4, 329 (1981).
12. Pimm, M.V., Jones, J.A., Price, M.R., Middle, J.G.,
    Embleton, M.J. and Baldwin, R.W.   Cancer Immunol.
    Immunother. 12, 125 (1982).
13. Rowland, G.F., Simmonds, R.G., Corvalan, J.R.F.,
    Baldwin, R.W., Brown, J.P., Embleton, M.J., Ford, C.H.J.,
    Hellstrom, K.E., Hellstrom, I., Kemshead, J.T.,
    Newman, C.F. and Woodhouse, C.S. 'Protides in Biological
    Fluids, Colloquium 30' (H. Peeters, ed.) p. 375.
    Pergamon Press, Oxford (1983).
14. Price, M.R., Pimm, M.V. and Baldwin, R.W. Br. J. Cancer
    44, 601 (1982).
15. Embleton, M.J., Pimm, M.V. and Baldwin, R.W. In 'Basic
    Mechanisms and Clinical Treatment of Tumour Metastases'

QUESTIONS AND ANSWERS

SCHLOM: The tissue localization seemed to show about a 2:1
(tumor: nontumor) specific localization, yet with the vindesine
therapy you showed a good effect. Why do you think it worked
so well?

BALDWIN: I agree that the localization data does not look the
best, but nonetheless it does bring a sufficient amount of
drug to the tumor for a therapeutic effect. Of course we are
looking for new antibodies with higher tumor-specific localization.

SUN: Does the conjugation of interferon to the monoclonal
antibody also reduce the biological activation of the attached
interferon molecules?

BALDWIN: Since the interferon is expected to activate natural
killer cells, we have not taken these studies very far.

IN VITRO SCREENING OF NEW MONOCLONAL
ANTI-CARCINOEMBRYONIC ANTIGEN ANTIBODIES
FOR RADIOIMAGING HUMAN COLORECTAL CARCINOMAS

Charles M. Haskell

Cancer Center, Medical Research Services
VA West Los Angeles
Department of Medicine, UCLA School of Medicine
Los Angeles, California

Franz Buchegger

Department of Biochemistry
University of Lausanne, Switzerland

Magali Schreyer, Stefan Carrel and Jean-Pierre Mach

Ludwig Institute for Cancer Research
Epalinges Sur/Lausanne, Switzerland

I. INTRODUCTION

Any form of passive immunotherapy for cancer, using either
native antibodies or antibodies as carriers of drugs, toxins,
or isotopes presupposes that the injected antibodies are
capable of localizing in their tumor cell target. We,
therefore, consider it essential to determine the capacity of
any antibody considered for immunotherapy to localize in
tumors in vivo. This can be tested in nude mice xenografted
with human cancer or in patients with cancer by injecting a
small amount of antibody labeled with ^{131}I and by observing
its distribution with external photoscanning. Such
immunoscintigraphic studies may have some diagnostic value for

cancer detection, but we consider them even more important for the selection of potential antibodies for passive immunotherapy.

Purified polyclonal antibodies against carcinoembryonic antigen (CEA) (1) have been shown by immunoscintigraphy to localize in human carcinomas, both in experimental animals (2,3) and in patients (4-6). However, only a single anti-CEA monoclonal antibody has been extensively tested and shown to concentrate in colorectal carcinoma tissue in patients (5,6). In this report we describe the screening and selection of anti-CEA monoclonal antibodies for studies of in vivo tumor localization.

II. MATERIALS AND METHODS

Balb/c mice were immunized intraperitoneally with 15µg of purified CEA in complete Freund's adjuvant on two occasions 3-1/2 months apart. One day after the second injection, mice received 100µg CEA intraperitoneally in saline, and one day later 150µg CEA in saline. Immunized mouse spleen cells were fused three days later with mouse myeloma NS1/1.AG 4.1 cells using 40% (v/v) polyethylene glycol, as described previously (7). Culture fluids of growing hybridomas were tested for the presence of anti-CEA antibody by a modification of the Farr assay, as described (7). Hybridomas producing antibody were cloned by limiting dilution, and subsequent studies of monoclonal antibody function were done with either hybridoma supernatants or purified antibody obtained from ascites collected from pristane-primed mice bearing hybridomas.

III. RESULTS AND DISCUSSION

A single fusion resulted in 26 hybridomas secreting antibodies binding to CEA. Because of the large number of positive hybridomas, it was impossible to clone them all initially; instead, preliminary immunochemical studies were performed to help guide the selection process and to provide comparative data with three monoclonal antibodies developed previously (7,8). The findings of these preliminary studies are presented in Table 1.

TABLE 1. Studies With Antibodies to CEA

Hybridoma Number	Tris versus PBS	Inhibition Studies		Immunoperoxidase	
		CEA	NCA	Colon Cancer	White Blood Cells
18	2.2	2.5	10,000	+	+
21	>3.0	1.6	4,000	+	±
35	1.5	1.6	40,000	+	−
54	0.5	>10.0	4,000	+	+
56	2.2	2.5	80,000	+	+
63	0.4	10.0	20,000	+	+
77	1.5	6.2	2,000	+	+
79	1.0	>10.0	4,000	+	±
100	>3.0	1.6	1,000	±	−
105	1.0	10.0	40	±	+
115	1.1	6.2	20,000	±	−
126	1.5	1.6	4,000	±	±
130	0	>10.0		±	−
131	2.0	10.0	10,000		
153	2.5	2.5	4,000	±	+
174	2.2	0.6	20,000	+	−
175	2.1	0.4	10,000	±	−
177	1.9	0.6	10,000	±	±
192	0.5	2.5	60	+	±
195	0.5			+	±
200	0.8	2.5	100	±	+
201	0.8	10.0	60	+	±
202	1.5	0.6	10,000	+	±
MAB					
23	3.0	2.5	60,000	+	±
47	1.5	>10.0	2,000	+	+
73	1.0	10.0	20,000	+	−

MAB = monoclonal antibody

The first results summarized in Table 1 represent a comparison of the ability of each supernatant to bind ^{125}I-labeled CEA in two different buffer systems. This was undertaken because monoclonal antibody 23, the original anti-CEA monoclonal antibody reported (7) and utilized in human studies (5,6), had been found to bind CEA much more efficiently in low molarity buffers than in physiologic saline, so it was postulated that a monoclonal antibody with better binding properties in physiologic saline might prove more effective in vivo. The studies were performed using the Farr assay with either 0.02M Tris HCl buffer pH 7.4 (low molarity) or 0.15M NaCl with 0.01M phosphate (PBS), pH 7.4 (physiologic molarity). Binding curves in PBS and Tris were compared and the antibody dilutions for PBS and Tris that gave 30% binding of CEA were determined. The figures in the second column of Table 1 indicate the difference in dilution (in log_{10}) between PBS and Tris to obtain the same binding of CEA. The titer of antibodies was always higher in 0.02M Tris. It can be seen that considerable differences in binding to soluble CEA exist between the various hybridoma supernatants tested in low and physiologic molarity buffers.

The third column in Table 1 shows the inhibition of binding to labeled CEA by preincubation of antibody with unlabeled CEA. This was undertaken to provide a preliminary assessment of the affinity of the antibodies (higher affinity being correlated with stronger inhibition of the monoclonal antibody by unlabeled CEA). Fourteen of the antibodies were inhibited by relatively small amounts of CEA (2.5 ng or less).

Inhibition of binding to labeled CEA by normal cross-reacting glycoprotein(s) (NCA or NGP) was studied at the same time as the studies of inhibition by unlabeled CEA. The results are expressed as the amounts of NCA (protein peak of 50 to 60,000 molecular weight from Sephadex G 200 filtration of perchloric acid extracts of normal lung) needed to achieve inhibition comparable to that seen with preincubation with unlabeled CEA. Thus, the higher the number, the lower the inhibition by NCA and the lower the quantitative cross-reactivity between the specificities recognized by the monoclonal antibodies and NCA. Based on these quantitative studies, the following antibody specificities were considered to have a relatively low cross-reactivity with NCA: 18,23,35,56,63,73,115,131,174,175,177,202.

The question of cross-reactivity with normal granulocytes was examined further by an immunoperoxidase technique on frozen tissue sections. The results of the indirect immunoperoxidase studies using tissue sections from human colon cancer are summarized in the last two columns of Table 1. This technique allows a visual distinction between the binding of hybridoma supernatants to colon cancer CEA on the apical side of tumor cells and the binding to NCA as seen in granulocytes infiltrating the basal layers of the tumor. Using this technique, hybridomas 35, 73 and 174 were of special interest since they bound CEA well but did not appear to bind to the NCA in normal granulocytes. All the other hybridomas reacted with moderate ($\pm$) or high (+) intensity to granulocytes infiltrating the tumor. After reviewing the results in Table 1, we chose to clone hybridomas 35, 192 and 202, and to study more intensively the monoclonal antibodies from these three hybridomas as well as monoclonal antibodies 23, 47 and 73.

In order to determine whether the new monoclonal antibodies reported here reacted with identical or with different antigenic determinants (epitopes) on the CEA molecule, radiolabeled (^{125}I or ^{131}I) monoclonal antibodies were tested for their binding capacity to CEA in a solid-phase radioimmunoassay, both with and without prior incubation with unlabeled monoclonal antibodies. In each case, complete inhibition of binding was obtained when the unlabeled, preincubated monoclonal antibody was the same as that of the radiolabeled monoclonal antibody. In addition, monoclonal antibodies 23 and 202 were completely cross-inhibitory and monoclonal antibodies 35 and 47 were partially cross-inhibitory. Monoclonal antibodies 192 and 73 were not inhibited by any of the other monoclonal antibodies. We interpret these results as suggesting a minimum of five epitopes for CEA, as recognized by our monoclonal antibodies, two of which are close to each other (epitopes for 35 and 47). Thus, monoclonal antibodies 23 and 202 identify the same or a spatially related epitope, while monoclonal antibodies 35, 47, 73 and 192 each identify separate epitopes.

The ability of these purified monoclonal antibodies to bind CEA in low molarity and physiologic molarity buffers was again tested, and the results summarized in Table 1 were confirmed. Similar studies were done with a direct binding assay using ^{125}I-labeled monoclonal antibodies and insolubilized CEA, and again the results were similar to those seen in the Farr assay in different buffer systems. We then directly tested the affinity (K_a) of monoclonal antibodies 23, 35, 192 and 202 by the method of Steward and Petty as described previously (7). The results of these direct measurements are shown in Table 2. Monoclonal antibody 23 had the highest affinity for CEA of the entire group when tested in low molarity buffer, however all three of the new monoclonal antibodies had higher K_a values than monoclonal antibody 23 when tested in physiologic saline.

TABLE 2.   Antibody Affinity

Monoclonal Antibody	Ka (liters/mole)	
	Low Molarity Buffer	Physiologic Buffer
23	6.0×10^{10}	5.7×10^{8}
35	1.6×10^{10}	5.6×10^{9}
192	2.3×10^{10}	1.8×10^{10}
202	4.4×10^{10}	1.1×10^{9}

Because of the importance of cross-reactivity with normal granulocyte glycoprotein(s), we tested the binding of monoclonal antibodies to ^{125}I-labeled NCA in a direct binding assay using the Farr assay. Monoclonal antibodies 23,35,47,73 and 202 did not react significantly with NCA, whereas an unabsorbed rabbit antiserum to CEA and monoclonal antibody 192 gave a very strong reaction.

The ability of monoclonal antibodies 23, 35, 192 and 202 to localize xenografts of human colon carcinoma in nude mice was then tested.   Nude mice bearing xenografts of human colon cancer CO-112 maintained by serial transplantation for many years were pretreated for four days with Lugol's solution and then injected intravenously with 5µg of freshly prepared ^{131}I-labeled purified monoclonal antibodies to CEA (dose of injected radioactivity 200µCi) together with 5µg of ^{125}I-labeled mouse IgG from myeloma P3X63 (dose of radioactivity 75µCi) as described (2,5). Total body scans were obtained three days later with a Picker thyroid scanning unit.   The tumor and normal organs were removed surgically after sacrificing the animal by ether anesthesia four days after injection.   The ^{131}I and ^{125}I radioactivity were determined in a dual channel gamma counter.

The best scans were obtained with monoclonal antibody 202, and the greatest specificity of localization expressed either as tumor uptake or as a specificity index was seen with this monoclonal antibody. Figure 1 demonstrates the scan achieved with monoclonal antibody 202, and Figure 2 shows the relative uptake of radiolabeled monoclonal antibody 202 or normal IgG in tumor and normal organs as measured in two mice.

In this study, monoclonal antibody 202 performed especially well in vitro and in the nude mouse model. It gave scan and tumor uptake values that were superior to monoclonal

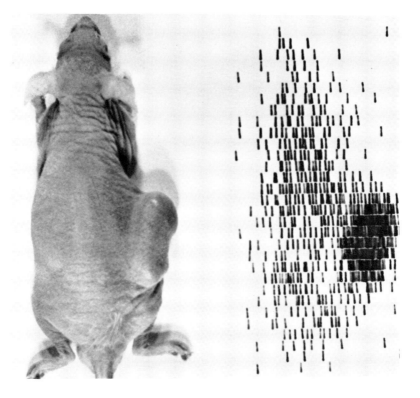

FIGURE 1. Nude mouse injected with ^{131}I-monoclonal antibody 202 and photoscan taken three days after injection.

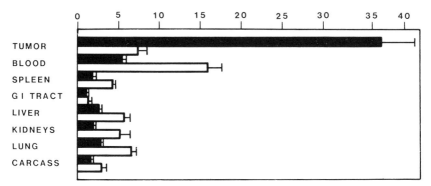

PERCENT CPM PER GRAM (mean + S.E.M.)

FIGURE 2. ^{131}I-monoclonal antibody 202 (black bars) versus ^{125}I-IgG (open bars) in tumor and normal tissue as percent total radioactivity four days after injection.

antibody 23, which is the monoclonal antibody used previously for immunoscintigraphy in humans (5,6). Since it appears that monoclonal antibody 202 is reacting against the same epitope on CEA as monoclonal antibody 23, it is likely that this improved performance relates to the fact that monoclonal antibody 202 has a higher affinity and better binding of CEA in physiologic solutions than does monoclonal antibody 23. It remains to be established whether monoclonal antibody 202 or one of the other new monoclonal antibodies to CEA taken individually or in a selected mixture will improve the results of immunoscinitigraphy using monoclonal antibody 23 in man. Similarly, further studies are necessary to clarify the predictive value of such screening studies in selecting monoclonal antibodies for human use.

ABBREVIATIONS

CEA, carcinoembryonic antigen; PBS, phosphate-buffered saline; NCA, normal cross-reacting antigen.

REFERENCES

1. Gold, P. and Freedman, S.O.   J. Exp. Med. 121, 439 (1965).
2. Mach, J-P., Carrel, S., Merenda, C., Sordat, B. and Cerottini, J-C. Nature 248, 704 (1974).
3. Goldenberg, D.M., Preston, D.F., Primus, F.J. and Hansen, H.J. Cancer Res. 34, 1 (1974).
4. Goldenberg, D.M., Kim E.E., DeLand, F.H., Bennett, S. and Primus, F.J. Cancer Res. 40, 2984 (1980).
5. Mach, J-P., Buchegger, F., Forni, M., Rischard, J., Berche, C., Lumbroso, J-D., Schreyer, M., Girardet, C., Accolla, R. and Carrel,S. Immunol. Today 2, 239 (1981).
6. Berche, C., Mach, J-P., Lumbroso, J-D., Langlais, C., Aubry, F., Buchegger, F., Carrel, S., Rougier, P., Parmentier, C. and Tubiana, M. Brit. Med. J. 285, 1447 (1982).
7. Accolla, R.S., Carrel, S. and Mach, J-P. Proc. Natl. Acad. Sci. USA 77, 563 (1980).
8. Buchegger, F., Mettraux, C., Accolla, R.S., Carrel, S. and Mach, J.P. Immunol. Letts. 5, 85 (1982).

QUESTIONS AND ANSWERS

MITCHELL: What is your control procedure to determine where the true tumor metastases are located? Some of the 'non-specific' localization may represent tumor deposits more sensitively detected by the radiolabeled monoclonal antibody.

MACH: Several of our patients were operated on after injection of labeled monoclonal antibody, and we could confirm that the increased concentration of radioactivity was in the tumor. For the unoperated patients, we had to rely on conventional methods of diagnosis.

RITZ: Can you give us some idea of the resolving power of this technique in terms of the smallest tumor you can detect?

MACH: We have detected as low as 3.6 grams of a medullary thyroid carcinoma, and at present we are not convinced that our present method can go lower than this. However, future improvements, particularly with indium labeling, may allow us to go below this size.

MONOCLONAL ANTIBODIES THAT BIND TO NORMAL AND NEOPLASTIC BREAST EPITHELIAL CELLS DISTINGUISH SUBSETS OF NORMAL BREAST EPITHELIAL CELLS

Paul A. W. Edwards and Christopher S. Foster

Ludwig Institute for Cancer Research (London Branch)
Royal Marsden Hospital
Sutton, Surrey, United Kingdom

I. INTRODUCTION

Recent work (1,2) with our panel of mouse monoclonal antibodies that bind to breast epithelial cells (3,4) has shown
that the antibodies distinguish at least three subsets of
breast lumenal epithelial cells. This is unexpected as, by
classical histology, these cells appear to be a homogeneous
population. Apart from the opportunities this observation
gives us to explore cell lineages and differentiation in the
breast, it could alter our approach to the selection of antibodies for diagnostic and therapeutic applications by throwing
new light on the problem of 'antigenic heterogeneity' in
tumors. The theme of this presentation is that cells in normal tissue show 'antigenic heterogeneity'; and, therefore, in
this respect tumors are only expressing a normal property of
their tissue of origin. The consequences of this for the
design of diagnostic and therapeutic antibodies will be
explored.

The monoclonal antibodies (LICR-LON-M8, LICR-LON-M18, and
LICR-LON-M24) were raised by essentially conventional methods
(3,5) using mice that had been immunized with human milk fat
globule membrane. The normal breast consists of branching
tubes of epithelium embedded in fibrous and fatty tissue. The
epithelium contains at least two types of cells, an outer
myoepithelial cell with contractile properties in the lactating state and a lumenal epithelial cell with the ability to

secrete milk. Within the breast, the monoclonal antibodies
bind specifically to the apical face of the lumenal epithelial
cells and do not bind to the surrounding myoepithelial cells,
connective tissue or blood vessel cells. They are not
breast-specific, as they react with some other epithelia (3).

II. ANTIGENIC HETEROGENEITY IN TUMORS

Most monoclonal antibodies that bind to cells in solid
tumors are found to bind to only some of the cells in a given
tumor (4,6-9). Different antibodies may bind to different
cells. Thus, a tumor is a heterogenous mixture of cells with
different surface antigens. Although it has been known for
some time that tumor cells are heterogeneous in several
respects (10,11), monoclonal antibodies have highlighted the
phenomenon; and, clearly, this hetergeneity appears to pose
serious problems for antibody therapy of tumors if any given
antibody will only bind to some of the tumor cells.

Our three monoclonal antibodies bind to both normal and
neoplastic breast epithelial cells. When they are used to
stain tumors, the heterogeneity of antigen expression is
clearly seen: the antibodies stain only some (or none) of the
cells in a tumor, and staining of serial sections shows that
the antibodies are often picking out different populations of
tumor cells. In particular, we (4 and unpublished observations) found that antibody LICR-LON-M8 often stains cells
around small lumina in tumors, whereas antibody LICR-LON-M24
stains cells in solid masses of tumor not adjacent to the
lumina. Thus, at least in some tumors, the different populations of cells stained by the different antibodies seem to be
in different physical environments in the tumor.

III. ANTIGENIC HETEROGENEITY IN NORMAL TISSUE

When used to stain normal intact breast tissue (1,2), it
was found that the three different monoclonal antibodies bind
to different subsets of normal lumenal epithelial cells. The
most elegant way to demonstrate the subsets of epithelial
cells distinguished by these antibodies, and to show how they
are arranged in two dimensions over the sheet of epithelium,
is to dissect out ducts from the normal breast, cut them open
with fine dissecting scissors and lay the epithelial sheet

flat. The apical faces of the unfixed and viable cells can
then be stained by the antibodies using immunofluorescence.
Figure 1 shows an example in which the subset of cells stained
by one antibody is compared with that stained by another using
two-color immunofluorescence. Figure 1(a) shows staining by
antibody M8 in fluorescein fluorescence; 1(b) shows antibody
M24 staining the same field in rhodamine fluorescence. M8
stains individual cells scattered over the epithelial pave-
ment; M24 stains a portion of the remaining cells. The arrows
mark the same cell in the two photographs; and, as color
photographs of this field show (1), the cells stained by antibody M8 are not stained by M24 and vice versa. This staining
pattern is typical, but there is some variation between
samples. M8 sometimes stains small groups of cells rather
than isolated cells, and staining by antibody M24 is often
more extensive, staining virtually all the cells left
unstained by antibody M8. The third antibody, M18, stains a
distinct subset of cells: usually less abundant, single cells
or small patches (1; not shown). Staining by the antibodies
can overlap (i.e., cells can be stained by more than one antibody).

IV. THESE OBSERVATIONS CAN BE GENERALIZED TO OTHER TISSUES AND MONOCLONAL ANTIBODIES.

Monoclonal antibodies raised in other laboratories
probably show similar properties. For example, Taylor-
Papdimitriou and her colleagues (6,14) noted that their two
monoclonal antibodies to breast epithelial cells bind to a
subset or subsets of normal epithelial cells. It seems likely
that other epithelia also consist of subsets of epithelial
cells expressing different surface phenotypes. When fresh
biopsies of the bladder are stained by antibodies M8 and M24
using two-color immunofluorescence (as in Figure 1), the two
antibodies pick out distinct subsets of the epithelial cells
(P.A.W. Edwards, I.M. Brooks and R.D. Pocock, unpublished
observations). Similarly, in fixed sections of the small
intestine, antibody M8 only stains some of the epithelial
cells (3).

V. INTERPRETATION AND CONSEQUENCES

Thus, surface antigenic heterogeneity is a property of normal tissue as well as tumors. In normal tissues, notably the hematopoietic system, cells expressing different surface antigens are generally in different states of differentiation (5,12,13). As yet we have no hard evidence that the different subsets of epithelial cells are in different states of differentiation, but it is an attractive idea supported by some circumstantial evidence. For example, in tumors there sometimes seems to be a correlation between antigenic phenotype and the position of cells in the tumor (see above); and, in primary cultures of normal breast, there seems to be a difference between the behavior of cells stained by antibody M18 and those stained by antibody M8 or M24 (1). One could imagine, for example, that cells stained by antibody M8 in the normal tissue could be mature secretory cells and those stained by M24 are in a quiescent state as far as secretion is concerned. This would parallel the presence of active and inactive cells seen in ultrastructural studies of lactating breast (15).

If antigenic phenotype is a reflection of normal differentiation, it is likely that the biological properties of tumor cells expressing the various antigens may be different; and, in particular, there is a possibility that one antigenic

FIGURE 1. Two-color immunofluorescence staining of intact, unfixed breast epithelium by monoclonal antibodies M8 and M24, looking down on the apical (lumenal) surface of the epithelial cells. X 280: scale can be gauged from (a) where individual cells are stained. (a) and (b) same piece of tissue; (a) staining by antibody M8 (fluorescein fluorescence); (b) staining by antibody M24 (rhodamine fluorescence). Staining procedures have been described elsewhere (1,2). Briefly, the tissue was incubated with the monoclonal antibodies followed by fluorescently labeled secondary antibodies; for M8 a goat anti-mouse (IgG1 subclass) fluorescein conjugate was used; for M24 an IgM-specific rhodamine conjugate was used.

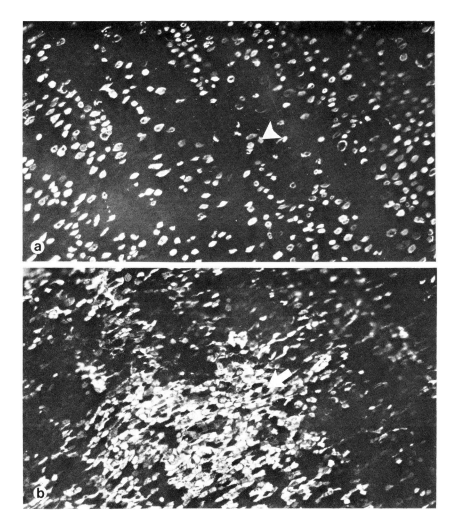

phenotype has greater potential for extended division or metastatic growth than the others. If so, it will be necessary,
in developing antibodies for possible therapy of tumors, to
raise and choose antibodies that recognize that population of
cells. Antibody-mediated destruction of the other populations
of tumor cells may have little effect on long-term growth. On
the other hand, when choosing antibodies for diagnostic procedures, such as detecting breast tumor cells in bone marrow
aspirates (16), it may be best to use an antibody or mixture
of antibodies that binds to most of the tumor cells rather
than a proliferating subset, as the latter may be too scarce
for efficient detection.

As antigenic heterogeneity is observed with many of the
monoclonal antibodies in current use, it is important to use
staining methods rather than bulk assays to determine the
distribution of the antigen. Cell lines also show antigenic
heterogeneity (1,8,14). To our knowledge, no antibody has yet
been described that has specificity for epithelial cells and
also has been shown unequivocally to bind to all the
epithelial cells in a particular tissue. The possibility that
antigenic phenotype reflects differentiation raises some
interesting questions. For example, are the tumor-associated
antigens described by Colcher et al. (7) expressed by some
rare types of normal breast epithelial cell, perhaps precursor
or stem cells? In radioimmune binding assays, melanoma cell
lines have been found to express various antigens to various
degrees (17). Is this because the melanoma lines have various
proportions of cells expressing particular antigenic phenotypes?

VI. CONCLUSION

The most important conclusion from this line of argument
for the development of therapeutic and diagnostic antibodies
is that it is possible that in a tumor the capacity for extensive proliferation is limited to a population of cells expressing a particular surface antigen. Antigenic heterogeneity
would then not be a bizarre obstacle to antibody therapy, but
merely a subtle reflection of biological complexity requiring
us to choose our antibody specificity with care.

ACKNOWLEDGMENTS

We thank Isobel Brooks, Elizabeth Dinsdale and Clare Smith for excellent assistance.

REFERENCES

1. Edwards, P.A.W. and Brooks, I.M. Differentiation, in press (1983).
2. Edwards, P.A.W. Biochem. Soc. Trans. 11:171 (1983).
3. Foster, C.S., Edwards, P.A.W., Dinsdale, E.A. and Neville, A.M. Virchows Arch. (Pathol. Anat.) 394, 279 (1982).
4. Foster, C.S., Dinsdale, E.A., Edwards, P.A.W. and Neville, A.M. Virchows Arch. (Pathol. Anat.) 394, 295 (1982).
5. Edwards, P.A.W. Biochem. J. 200, 1 (1981).
6. Arklie, J., Taylor-Papadimitriou, J., Bodmer, W., Egan, M. and Millis, R. Int. J. Cancer 28, 23 (1981).
7. Colcher, D., Horan-Hand, O., Nuti, M. and Schlom, J. Proc. Natl. Acad. Sci. USA 78, 3199 (1981).
8. Nuti, M., Teramoto, Y.A., Mariani-Costantini, R., Horan Hand, P., Colcher, D. and Schlom, J. Int. J. Cancer 29, 539 (1982).
9. McGee, J.O'D., Woods, J.C., Ashall, F., Bramwell, M.E. and Harris, H. Lancet, July 3, 7 (1982).
10. Miller, F.R. and Heppner, G.H. J. Natl. Cancer Inst. 63, 1457 (1979).
11. Kerbel, R.S. Nature (News and Views) 28, 358 (1979).
12. Williams, A.F., Galfre, G., Milstein, C. Cell 12, 663 (1977).
13. Boyse, E.A. and Old, L.J. Ann. Rev. Genet. 3, 269 (1969).
14. Chang, S.E., Keen, J., Lane, E.B. and Taylor-Papadimitriou, J. Cancer Res. 42, 2040 (1982).
15. Tobon, H. and Salazar, H. J. Clin. Endocrinol. Metab. 40, 834 (1974).
16. Dearnaley, D.P., Sloane, J.P., Ormerod, M.G., Steele, K., Coombes, R.C., Clink, H.M., Powles, T.J., Ford, H.T., Gazet, J-C., and Neville, A.M. Br. J. Cancer 44, 85 (1981).
17. Houghton, A.N., Eisinger, M., Albino, A.P., Cairncross, J.G. and Old, L.J. J. Exp. Med. 156, 1755 (1982).

QUESTIONS AND ANSWERS

THORPE: Are the antigens intracellular or extracellular?

EDWARDS: All are cell surface. They can be seen both before and after fixing.

MASON: You have presented a picture where the epithelial cells express one or another cell surface marker and therefore the duct is a mosaic of these different cell types. I wonder if you selected these antibodies because they show exclusive binding to one cell type.

EDWARDS: No. Of the antibodies we made, all show one of the three distinctive staining patterns I showed. Furthermore, we recently looked at some of the monoclonal antibodies made by Joyce Taylor-Papadimitriou using primary tissue culture cells and found them to behave similarly to one of the antibodies I described; however, we have not looked at freshly dissected duct as yet.

TAYLOR-PAPADIMITRIOU: Since many of these antibodies bind to similar molecules, it will be necessary to identify the antigenic determinants and look to see if this staining pattern is due to cells expressing variable forms of the antigen at different stages of differentiation.

EDWARDS: At this stage we know that one does not bind a high molecular weight glycoprotein while another does. The third binds to a simple sugar group found on several different glycoproteins.

MASON: Have you been able to isolate the three cell types as separate populations?

EDWARDS: Yes, the fluorescence-activated cell sorter can pick out the three populations.

MACH: You have three monoclonal antibodies raised against milk fat globule antigens, which appear to recognize three subpopulations of cells in the normal breast tubule. Among the breast carcinomas that you have tested, did you find some which reacted only with one or two of the three monoclonal antibodies?

EDWARDS: Every tumor is positive for the green antibody, which is very similar to the one we obtained from Joyce Taylor-Papadimitriou. About half of the tumors stain with the red antibody, and only a small proportion stain with the third antibody.

LENNOX: Since patterns of glycosolation on a single poly-peptide can be enormously variable and we have seen many very similar antibody binding patterns, like the carcinoembryonic antigen family, what is being done to fit the monoclonal anti-bodies into an overall scheme which might tell us when a glycosylation change has occurred as compared with a change in the polypeptides to which these are attached? For example, where does Ca1 fit into your scheme?

EDWARDS: I have collected antibodies from four different groups to start a comparison of fluorescence binding, and Dr. Taylor-Papadimitriou is looking at the chemistry.

LENNOX: Is Ca1 included in this study?

EDWARDS: No. However, it is planned for inclusion later.

TAYLOR-PAPADIMITRIOU: (Comment) In deciding whether the various antibodies to milk fat globule have a similar spectrum of reactivity when considered amongst themselves and with other antibodies, it is important to try to chemically identify the antigenic determinants. Where they are against carbohydrate determinants, they may react with the same molecule and block each other even if they are against different epitopes in the complex carbohydrate side chain. Blocking of staining pattern therefore has only limited usefulness in determining cross-reactions of antibodies with this type of specificity.

As a final step one can test whether the various antibodies to high molecular weight glycoproteins react with the same molecules using a combination of precipitation and blasting techniques. Whether they react with the same epitope requires chemical clarification of the oligosaccharide sequence.

Index

A

Adenocarcinomas, monoclonal antibodies and, 199–206

Adenomas, monoclonal antibodies and, 199–206

Adriamycin
and autologous bone marrow transplantation, 74–75
conjugated with monoclonal antibody, 273

Allogeneic bone marrow transplantation, 107–116
and anti-T cell immunotoxins, 90–92

Alpha-emitting isotope–monoclonal antibody conjugates, antitumor effects of, 128–131

Alpha fetoprotein, rat anti-mouse antibody to, 223–225

Antibody, monoclonal, *see* Monoclonal antibody

Antigenic determinants, cancer associated, *see also* specific determinants
and breast cancer, 228–230
and intestinal tract carcinomas, 235
and melanomas, 235

Antigenic expression, tumors and, 58, 66, *see also* Antigenic heterogeneity, specific tumors

Antigenic heterogeneity
in epithelial neoplasms, 188–191
in normal breast tissue, 285–292
in tumors of breast, 285–286, 292–293

Antigenic modulation
in humans receiving murine monoclonal antibodies, 10–11, 16, 49–50
and monoclonal antibodies to growth-related receptors, 58, 61

Antigens, cell surface, and glioma cell differentiation, 239–242, *see also* specific antigens

Anti-idiotype–A chain conjugates, and BCL$_1$ tumors in mice, 92–95

Anti-idiotype response, in humans receiving mouse monoclonal antibodies, 10, 12, 15, 16, 93, *see also* Tolerization

Anti-IgD immunotoxins, mouse B cell leukemia and, 92–93

Anti-Leu-1, 7–16

Anti-mouse Ig response, in humans receiving mouse monoclonal antibodies, 7–8, 10, 15–16, 28–33, 163

Anti-Thy1 antibodies
ricin-containing, 90
and SL-2 leukemia model, 55
and T cell leukemia, 63–71

Anti-Y 29/55, 74–78, 215–221

Aplastic anemia, and allogeneic bone marrow transplantation, 90–92

Autologous bone marrow transplantation (ABMT), 74–78, 85, 87–92
and *in vitro* purging of bone marrow with monoclonal antibodies, 74–78
with ricin–antibody conjugates, 87–90

B

B cell tumors, monoclonal antibody identification of, 198, 215–221

Benign prostatic hypertrophy, 167–170

Bladder epithelial cells, detection of subsets of, 287

B-leukemia-associated monoclonal antibody, 73–79

B lymphocytes
differentiation of, 215–216
monoclonal antibodies to, 215–221

Blocked conjugates, *see* Ricin
B non-Hodgkin's lymphoma, 74–78, 217
Bone marrow cells
    labeling, 42
    purging, *see* Autologous bone marrow
        transplantation
Brain tumor cells, differentiation of,
    239–242
Breast cancer, *see also* Human milk fat
        globule
    and human milk fat globule, 227–238
    and Ia-like antigens, 246–250
    monoclonal antibodies reactive against,
        199–200, 207–208
Breast epithelial cells, detection of subsets
    of, 285–293

C

Carbohydrate antigens, cancer associated,
    see Gastrointestinal cancer antigen,
    Lacto-*N*-fucopentaose II,
    Lacto-*N*-fucopentaose III
Carcinoembryonic antigen (CEA), 17
    and colorectal carcinoma, 34–35,
        199–206
    and epithelial tumors, 188–190, 194
    and imaging of tumors, 275–283
    and localization of tumors, 276–283
    and nonneoplastic cells, 190–194
Carcinoma, human, *see also* specific
        carcinomas
    antigenic cross-reactivity among, 199
    monoclonal antibody reactivity and,
        199–206
Cervix, tumors of, 164–170
Chamber, diffusion, for monoclonal
    antibody administration, 172–180
Chemotherapy, *see* specific drugs
Colitis, ulcerative, 201–206
Colorectal cancer, 171, *see also*
        Carcinoembryonic antigen,
        Gastrointestinal cancer antigen
    and gastrointestinal cancer antigen, 19
    and HMFG-2, 234
    imaging, 268, 270, 275–283
    and lacto-*N*-fucopentaose II, 251
    and lacto-*N*-fucopentaose III, 255–258,
        260
    and Lewis blood group, 252, 255–258
    reactivity of monoclonal antibodies and,
        199–206
    treatment, 28–35
Complement, 12, 24, 38, 74–78, 90

Conjugates, cytocidal agent–monoclonal
        antibody, therapeutic effects of,
        127–131, *see also* Drug targeting,
        Immunotoxins, Ricin–antibody
        conjugates
Cyclophosphamide
    and anti-mouse Ig antibody response in
        humans, 7
    and autologous bone marrow
        transplantation, 74–75
    and spontaneous leukemia in mice,
        67–71
Cytokeratin intermediate filament
    determinant, 193

D

Desmin, 192
Diagnosis, of tumors, monoclonal antibodies
    in, 171, 192–198, 208–213, *see also*
    Imaging, Localization
Differentiation, cellular, of tumors, 192,
    229–236, 239–242, 288–289, 292, *see
    also* specific tumors
Diphtheria toxin, 110–112, 122, 128,
    130–131
Drug targeting, 268–274, *see also* specific
    agents, Localization

E

Effector cells, 24–25, 71
Epidermal growth factor receptor, 58–59
Epithelia-associated antigens, and cancer,
    188–198
Epstein–Barr virus
    in humans receiving monoclonal
        antibodies, 179
    and hybridomas, 135, 137, 144, 162, 166
Erythroid burst-forming unit, immunotoxins
    and, 89
Erythroid colony-forming unit,
    immunotoxins and, 89

F

Fusing partners, *see* Monoclonal antibody
    production

G

Gastrointestinal tract cancer, 17–21, *see
    also* Colorectal cancer

Gastrointestinal cancer antigen (GICA), 18–20, 25–28, *see also* Lacto-*N*-fucopentaose II, Lacto-*N*-fucopentaose III
Glial cell tumors, 239–242
Glial fibrillary acidic protein, 192
Glioma
  antibody diffusion chamber and, 172
  localization, 175–178
Graft-versus-host disease, *see* Allogeneic bone marrow transplantation

H

Hematopoietic colony-forming cells, immunotoxin effect on, 89
Hepatocarcinoma, 223
Heteromyeloma, *see* Hybridoma, mouse–human
HLA-DR antigens, 188–191, 197, 243–250
Human milk fat globule (HMFG), 285
  antigenic determinants of, 228–230
  and breast cancer, 227–238
  and preinvasive breast lesions, 238
Hybridomas, human–human
  cell lines used in production of, 143–155
  development of, 136, 143–155, 157–162, 181–184
  monoclonal antibody production by, 164–170
Hybridomas, mouse–human, 135–142, 164–170
Hybridomas, mouse–mouse, 135

I

Ia-like antigens, 244–250
I blood group, 232
Imaging, with monoclonal antibodies, 22, 23, 125–127, 130–131, 267–268, 276–283, *see also* Localization
Immunohistological analysis of human tumors, 187–198
Immunoscintigraphy, *see* Imaging, Localization
Immunotoxins, 85–98, 99–106, 107–116, 117–124, 125–131, *see also* Conjugates, Ricin
Insulin receptor, 58–59
Interleukin 2 receptor, 58–59
Interferon, 268, 272–273, 274

K

Keratin-associated antigens, 188–190, 193, 197

Kidney, tumors of, 164–170

L

Lactating breast cells, differentiation antigens of, 229–230
Lacto-*N*-fucopentaose II, 251–255
Lacto-*N*-fucopentaose III, 255–258, 260
Leukemia
  acute lymphoblastic, 7–12, 74
  and allogeneic bone marrow transplantation, 108
  and autologous bone marrow transplantation, 74–78
  chronic lymphocytic, 40, 42–46, 74–78
  hairy cell, 74–78, 217
  spontaneous, in mice, 66–71
  treatment of, 7–12, 39–46, 48–50, 54–59, 63–71, 87–98, 101–106, 127–131
  T cell, 63–71, 101–106, 166–170
Leukocyte-common antigen, 192
Lewis blood group
  and colorectal cancer, 255
  and gastrointestinal cancer antigen, 21
  and lacto-*N*-fucopentaose II, 252
  and lacto-*N*-fucopentaose III, 255–258, 260
  Le^a antigen, 19, 21
  Le^b antigen, 21, 25–28, 255
  Le^x antigen, 25–28
Localization, tumor, 15, 48, 234–235, 238, 266–270, 274, 275, 276–283
Lung, cancer of
  antigenic determinants associated with, 165–170
  localization, 178
Lymphoid neoplasms, antigens of, 188–190
Lymphoma
  and autologous bone marrow transplantation, 74–78
  treatment of, 7–12, 40, 44–48, 119–123, 171, 217

M

Macrophages, 24–25, 197
Magic bullet, *see* Drug targeting, Localization, specific conjugates
Mammary cancer, *see* Breast cancer
Melanoma, human, 101–106
Metastases, *see also* Transforming factors
  antigenic variation in, 25–28, 66
  detection, 23, 208, 283

Methotrexate—monoclonal antibody
conjugate, 271–272
Modulation, antigenic, see Antigenic
modulation
Monoclonal antibodies, see also specific
antigens and antibodies
administration via diffusion chamber,
172–180
antitumor effects, 12
conjugated with cytocidal agents, 87–89,
127–131, 268–274
and diagnosis of tumors, 171, 192–198,
208–213
human, vs. murine, 163, 171–172
toxicity of, 6, 50, 57, 70–71
tumor specificity of, 190, 192–198,
207–213
Monoclonal antibody production, 135–142,
143–155, 157–162, 171–180,
181–184, see also Hybridomas
fusing partners, 143–155
Murine monoclonal antibodies, see also
Monoclonal antibodies
anti-Leu-1, 7–16
anti-Thy1.1, 63–71
anti-human transferrin, 261–264
anti-transferrin receptor, 53–61
anti-Y 29/55, 73–79
to gastrointestinal cancer antigen, 17–38
T101, 40–52

N

Neuroblastoma antigen, 192
Neuronal cell tumors, 239–242
Non-Hodgkin's lymphoma, 73–78

O

Ovary, cancer of, 207–210, 211–213, 234

P

Pancreas, cancer of, 19
Pluripotential stem cells, 89
Prednisone, and autologous bone marrow
transplantation, 74
Preinvasive lesions, detection of, 238
Proliferation, cellular, in tumors
and antigen expression, 290
and treatment, 53–61
Prostate, carcinoma of, 164–170

R

Rabbit anti-Ig—A-chain conjugate, 87–89

Radiation therapy
and autologous bone marrow
transplantation, 75, 77
and colorectal cancer, 33–35
Rat anti-mouse monoclonal antibodies,
55–61, 223–225
Ricin, see also Ricin-antibody conjugates
and autologous bone marrow
transplantation, 85–98
galactose-binding site, blockade of,
117–124
toxicity of, and A chain, 100
Ricin—antibody conjugates
A chain—antibody conjugates, 99–106
and allogeneic bone marrow
transplantation, 107–116
anti-Thy1.1—ricin conjugate, 118–124
disulphide bond and, 100, 103, 117, 123
galactose-binding site and, 117–124
half life of, 131
thioether bond and, 103, 123
toxicity, 110, 120, 122
W3/25—ricin conjugate, 118–124

S

S-100 protein, 192
Sarcoma, osteogenic, 265–274
drug targeting, 268–273, 274
imaging, 267–268, 269
localization, 266–267
Sialyl-lacto-N-pentaosyl II ganglioside, 17
Stage-specific embryonic antigen, 257
Stomach, cancer of, 19, see also
Gastrointestinal cancer
Surgical treatment, monoclonal antibody
therapy and, 33–35

T

T65 antigen, 42
Targeting, tumor, see Imaging
T cell killing, ricin—antibody conjugates
and, 107–116
T cell lymphoma, cutaneous, 7–12, 40,
44–48
Teratocarcinoma, 223
Thymomas, 197
Thyroid carcinoma, detection of, 283
Tissue processing, effect of, on antigenic
determinants, 192–196
Tolerization, 16, 33, 93–95
Toxicity, of monoclonal antibodies, 6, 49,
50, 57, 70–71, see also specific
antibodies and conjugates

Transferrin
  binding of monoclonal antibodies to,
    263–264
  interaction with transferrin receptor,
    262–263
Transferrin receptor
  in human cutaneous basal cell carcinoma,
    188–198
  monoclonal antibodies to, 53–61
Transforming factors, tumor progression
    and, in cells, 61
Tumor-associated antigens, 153–155,
    163–170, 187–198, 199–206,
    207–213, 215–221, 223–225,
    227–238, 239–242, 243–249,
    251–260, *see also* Imaging,
    Localization, specific antigens and
    tumors
Tumors, heterotransplanted human, study
    of, 21–25

U

Uterine adenocarcinoma, 193, 197–198

V

Vimentin, 192, 197–198
Vincristine, and autologous bone marrow
    transplantation, 74–75
Vindesine–antibody conjugate, 268–271

W

White blood cell count, monoclonal
    antibody administration and, 67–71

Y

Y 29/55 antigen, 74–78, 215–221